PHARMACY
CALCULATION
WORKBOOK

ISBN: 1733837744
ISBN-13: 978-1733837743

CONTENTS

SECTION 1

CALCULATION FUNDAMENTALS

QUESTIONS

1. Calculate how many milliliters of Maalox a patient will receive in each dose of the following prescription.

   Rx:
   Benadryl 12.5 mg/5 mL   80 mL
   Lidocaine 2%   30 mL
   Maalox   qs ad 200 mL
   Sig: i tbsp po tid

   a. 4.5 mL
   b. 6.75 mL
   c. 7.25 mL
   d. 8.75 mL

2. Calculate how many milliliters must be dispensed for the following prescription.

   Rx:
   Amoxicillin 400 mg/5 mL
   Sig: ii tsp po q8h × 10 days

   a. 250 mL
   b. 280 mL
   c. 300 mL
   d. 330 mL

3. A patient is dispensed a 10 milliliter vial of insulin that contains 100 units/mL. How many days will the vial last if the patient uses 50 units per day?

   a. 20 days
   b. 25 days
   c. 28 days
   d. 30 days

4. A patient is to receive 10 doses of azithromycin 250 mg. If the pharmacy has one gram vials available, how many vials will need to be used to prepare the 10 doses? (Round answer to the nearest whole number.)

   a. 2 vials
   b. 3 vials
   c. 4 vials
   d. 6 vials

5. A patient is to receive 2 teaspoons of sucralfate every 6 hours. How many milliliters per day will the patient receive?

a. 20 mL
b. 25 mL
c. 32 mL
d. 40 mL

6. Calculate how many tablets are needed to fill the following prescription.

Rx:
Furosemide 20 mg
Sig: ii tabs po bid × 5 days

a. 20 tablets
b. 24 tablets
c. 28 tablets
d. 30 tablets

7. A 30 milliliter bottle of a nasal spray delivers 25 sprays per milliliter of solution. Each spray contains 2 milligrams of active medication. How many grams of the medication are contained in each 30 milliliter bottle?

a. 1.2 g
b. 1.5 g
c. 2.5 g
d. 2.8 g

8. Calculate how many doses are contained in the quantity dispensed for the following prescription.

Rx:
Amoxicillin 400 mg/5 mL
Dispense 100 mL
Sig: i tsp po bid

a. 8 doses
b. 10 doses
c. 20 doses
d. 25 doses

9. A patient is taking 2 teaspoons every 8 hours of cephalexin 250 mg/5 mL. How many milligrams of cephalexin is the patient receiving per day?

    a. 800 mg
    b. 900 mg
    c. 1200 mg
    d. 1500 mg

10. Calculate the days supply for the following prescription. (Assume 1 milliliter contains 15 drops of medication and round answer down to the nearest whole number.)

    Rx:
    Maxitrol Susp.
    Dispense 5 mL bottle
    Sig: 2 gtts os qid

    a. 5 days
    b. 7 days
    c. 9 days
    d. 10 days

11. How many milligrams of phenobarbital will a patient receive per day for the following prescription?

    Rx:
    Phenobarbital ½ gr
    Dispense 60 tabs
    Sig: i tab po bid

    a. 32 mg
    b. 65 mg
    c. 90 mg
    d. 120 mg

12. A vial of dexamethasone has a concentration of 4 mg/mL. How many milliliters would be given to a patient requiring a 10 milligram dose?

    a. 2.5 mL
    b. 3 mL
    c. 4.5 mL
    d. 5 mL

13. Calculate how many capsules are needed to fill the following prescription.

Rx:
Fluoxetine 10 mg
Dispense 60 day supply
Sig: 3 caps po qam

a. 90 capsules
b. 180 capsules
c. 270 capsules
d. 360 capsules

14. A cough syrup contains 6 milligrams of dextromethorphan per milliliter of solution. How many milligrams of dextromethorphan are in two teaspoons?

a. 15 mg
b. 30 mg
c. 60 mg
d. 80 mg

15. A prescription calls for 20 mg/kg of vancomycin every 8 hours. How many milligrams of vancomycin will a patient weighing 80 kilograms receive per day?

a. 1600 mg
b. 2400 mg
c. 3200 mg
d. 4800 mg

16. Digoxin solution for injection is available in a concentration of 0.25 mg/mL. How many milliliters are needed for a 200 microgram dose of digoxin?

a. 0.8 mL
b. 1.3 mL
c. 1.9 mL
d. 2.2 mL

17. Calculate the days supply for the following prescription if an inhaler containing 200 puffs is dispensed.

Rx:
Albuterol sulfate 90 mcg/inhalation
Sig: 2 puffs q6h prn

a. 14 days
b. 20 days
c. 25 days
d. 30 days

18. A prescription calls for heparin 5000 units intravenously every 8 hours. Multi-dose vials are available that have a concentration of 10,000 units/mL. How many milliliters of heparin will be needed per day?

    a. 0.8 mL
    b. 1 mL
    c. 1.5 mL
    d. 1.75 mL

19. A patient is to receive 25 units of insulin glargine once daily at bedtime. How many milliliters will be used every day if a 10 milliliter vial contains 100 units/mL?

    a. 0.25 mL
    b. 0.4 mL
    c. 0.55 mL
    d. 0.7 mL

20. An ophthalmic solution of tobramycin has a concentration of 3 mg/mL. If an eyedropper is calibrated to deliver 16 drops per milliliter, how many milligrams of tobramycin would be contained in 2 drops?

    a. 0.375 mg
    b. 0.5 mg
    c. 0.825 mg
    d. 0.85 mg

21. How many milliliters per day will a patient use for the following prescription?

    Rx:
    Lactulose 10 g/15 mL
    Sig: ii tbsp po bid × 5 days

    a. 20 mL
    b. 30 mL
    c. 40 mL
    d. 60 mL

22. A prescriber orders 750 mg tablets of ciprofloxacin to be taken twice a day for 5 days. How many total grams of ciprofloxacin are prescribed?

    a. 4 g
    b. 6.5 g
    c. 7.5 g
    d. 8 g

23. Calculate how many tablets are needed to fill the following prescription.

Rx:
Prednisone 20 mg
Sig: 3 tabs po qd × 3 days, 2 tabs po qd × 3 days, 1 tab po qd × 3 days

a. 16 tablets
b. 18 tablets
c. 22 tablets
d. 26 tablets

24. A patient is to receive 2 grams of cefazolin every 8 hours. The pharmacy has a 20 milliliter vial that has a concentration of 1000 mg/5 mL. How many milliliters are needed per dose?

a. 2.5 mL
b. 5 mL
c. 7.5 mL
d. 10 mL

25. A patient is to receive an intravenous infusion of 40 milliequivalents per hour of potassium chloride. How many milliequivalents of potassium chloride are administered every minute?

a. 0.42 mEq
b. 0.55 mEq
c. 0.67 mEq
d. 0.84 mEq

ANSWER KEY

1. B
Step 1: Calculate the quantity of Maalox required for the prescription.
200 mL – (80 mL + 30 mL) = 90 mL

Step 2: Calculate how many milliliters of Maalox will be in each dose.

a. $\dfrac{90 \text{ mL}}{200 \text{ mL}} = \dfrac{x \text{ mL}}{15 \text{ mL}}$

b. $200x = 1350$

c. $x = 6.75 \text{ mL}$

2. C

$\dfrac{10 \text{ mL}}{\text{dose}} \times \dfrac{3 \text{ doses}}{\text{day}} \times 10 \text{ days} = 300 \text{ mL}$

3. A

$10 \text{ mL} \times \dfrac{100 \text{ units}}{1 \text{ mL}} \times \dfrac{1 \text{ day}}{50 \text{ units}} = 20 \text{ days}$

4. B
Step 1: 0.25 g × 10 doses = 2.5 g
Step 2: 2.5 g × 1 vial/g = 2.5 vials = 3 vials

5. D

$\dfrac{2 \text{ tsp}}{\text{dose}} \times \dfrac{4 \text{ doses}}{\text{day}} \times \dfrac{5 \text{ mL}}{1 \text{ tsp}} = 40 \text{ mL/day}$

6. A

$\dfrac{2 \text{ tabs}}{\text{dose}} \times \dfrac{2 \text{ doses}}{\text{day}} \times 5 \text{ days} = 20 \text{ tablets}$

7. B
Step 1: Calculate how many grams of medication are in each milliliter of solution.

$\dfrac{2 \text{ mg}}{1 \text{ spray}} \times \dfrac{1 \text{ g}}{1000 \text{ mg}} \times \dfrac{25 \text{ sprays}}{1 \text{ mL}} = 0.05 \text{ g/mL}$

Step 2: Calculate how many grams of medication are in a 30 milliliter bottle.
0.05 g/mL × 30 mL = 1.5 g

8. C

$100 \text{ mL} \times \dfrac{1 \text{ dose}}{5 \text{ mL}} = 20 \text{ doses}$

9. D

$$\frac{10 \text{ mL}}{\text{dose}} \times \frac{3 \text{ doses}}{\text{day}} \times \frac{250 \text{ mg}}{5 \text{ mL}} = 1500 \text{ mg/day}$$

10. C

$$5 \text{ mL} \times \frac{15 \text{ gtts}}{1 \text{ mL}} \times \frac{1 \text{ day}}{8 \text{ gtts}} = 9.375 \text{ days} = 9 \text{ days}$$

11. B

$$\frac{0.5 \text{ gr}}{1 \text{ tab}} \times \frac{65 \text{ mg}}{1 \text{ gr}} \times \frac{1 \text{ tab}}{\text{dose}} \times \frac{2 \text{ doses}}{\text{day}} = 65 \text{ mg/day}$$

12. A

Step 1: $\dfrac{4 \text{ mg}}{1 \text{ mL}} = \dfrac{10 \text{ mg}}{x \text{ mL}}$

Step 2: $4x = 10$

Step 3: $x = 2.5 \text{ mL}$

13. B

60 days × 3 caps/day = 180 capsules

14. C

6 mg/mL × 10 mL = 60 mg

15. D

$$80 \text{ kg} \times \frac{20 \text{ mg}}{\text{kg/dose}} \times \frac{3 \text{ doses}}{\text{day}} = 4800 \text{ mg/day}$$

16. A

Step 1: $\dfrac{0.25 \text{ mg}}{1 \text{ mL}} = \dfrac{0.2 \text{ mg}}{x \text{ mL}}$

Step 2: $0.25x = 0.2$

Step 3: $x = 0.8 \text{ mL}$

17. C

$$200 \text{ puffs} \times \frac{1 \text{ dose}}{2 \text{ puffs}} \times \frac{1 \text{ day}}{4 \text{ doses}} = 25 \text{ days}$$

18. C

$$\frac{5000 \text{ units}}{\text{dose}} \times \frac{1 \text{ mL}}{10{,}000 \text{ units}} \times \frac{3 \text{ doses}}{\text{day}} = 1.5 \text{ mL/day}$$

19. A

$$\frac{1 \text{ mL}}{100 \text{ units}} \times \frac{25 \text{ units}}{\text{day}} = 0.25 \text{ mL/day}$$

20. A

$$2 \text{ gtts} \times \frac{1 \text{ mL}}{16 \text{ gtts}} \times \frac{3 \text{ mg}}{1 \text{ mL}} = 0.375 \text{ mg}$$

21. D

$$\frac{30 \text{ mL}}{\text{dose}} \times \frac{2 \text{ doses}}{\text{day}} = 60 \text{ mL/day}$$

22. C

$$\frac{750 \text{ mg}}{\text{dose}} \times \frac{1 \text{ g}}{1000 \text{ mg}} \times \frac{2 \text{ doses}}{\text{day}} \times 5 \text{ days} = 7.5 \text{ g}$$

23. B

(3 tabs/day × 3 days) + (2 tabs/day × 3 days) + (1 tab/day × 3 days) = 18 tablets

24. D

$$\frac{2 \text{ g}}{\text{dose}} \times \frac{1000 \text{ mg}}{1 \text{ g}} \times \frac{5 \text{ mL}}{1000 \text{ mg}} = 10 \text{ mL}$$

25. C

$$\frac{40 \text{ mEq}}{1 \text{ hr}} \times \frac{1 \text{ hr}}{60 \text{ min}} = 0.67 \text{ mEq/min}$$

SECTION 2

DENSITY AND SPECIFIC GRAVITY

QUESTIONS

1. Calculate the weight in grams of three liters of glycerin that has a density of 1.26 g/mL.

   a. 1853 g
   b. 2380 g
   c. 3476 g
   d. 3780 g

2. Calculate the number of milliliters of propylene glycol (SG = 1.03) required to prepare twelve 60 gram tubes of the following formula for a testosterone gel.

Testosterone powder, micronized	4 g
Propylene glycol	1 g
Methylcellulose 2% gel	55 g

   a. 1.94 mL
   b. 3.68 mL
   c. 7.25 mL
   d. 11.65 mL

3. Calculate the specific gravity of a quart of oil that weighs 720 grams.

   a. 0.48
   b. 0.76
   c. 0.93
   d. 1.52

4. Calculate the weight in grams of one pint of propylene glycol that has a specific gravity of 1.03.

   a. 450.1 g
   b. 459.2 g
   c. 487.2 g
   d. 496.3 g

5. A compound requires 5 grams of castor oil (SG = 0.96). How many milliliters of castor oil should be measured?

   a. 4.8 mL
   b. 5.2 mL
   c. 5.9 mL
   d. 6.1 mL

6. Calculate the total weight of the following formula for a topical preparation. The specific gravity of isopropyl alcohol is 0.78.

Hydrocortisone	0.6 g
Isopropyl alcohol	4.3 mL
Purified water	25.7 mL

a. 26.38 g
b. 29.65 g
c. 30.61 g
d. 39.74 g

7. Calculate the volume in liters of one pound of hydrochloric acid (SG = 1.37).

a. 0.33 L
b. 0.45 L
c. 0.51 L
d. 0.62 L

8. Calculate the density of one gallon of a liquid that weighs 568 grams.

a. 0.15 g/mL
b. 0.36 g/mL
c. 0.71 g/mL
d. 0.92 g/mL

9. A compound requires 8 milliliters of liquefied phenol (SG = 1.07). How many milligrams is this equivalent to?

a. 4238 mg
b. 7477 mg
c. 8560 mg
d. 9534 mg

10. Calculate the density of one liter of alcohol that weighs 978 grams.

a. 0.978 g/mL
b. 1.022 g/mL
c. 1.367 g/mL
d. 1.874 g/mL

ANSWER KEY

1. D
1.26 g/mL × 3000 mL = 3780 g

2. D
Step 1: Calculate how many grams of propylene glycol are required.
12 tubes × 1 g/tube = 12 g

Step 2: Calculate how many milliliters of propylene glycol are required.
12 g ÷ 1.03 = 11.65 mL

3. B
720 g ÷ 946 mL = 0.76

4. C
473 mL × 1.03 = 487.2 g

5. B
5 g ÷ 0.96 = 5.2 mL

6. B
Step 1: Calculate the number of grams of isopropyl alcohol.
4.3 mL × 0.78 = 3.354 g

Step 2: Calculate the number of grams of purified water.
25.7 mL × 1 = 25.7 g

Step 3: Calculate the total weight of the formula.
0.6 g + 3.354 g + 25.7 g = 29.65 g

7. A
454 g ÷ 1.37 = 331.4 mL ÷ 1000 = 0.33 L

8. A
568 g ÷ 3785 mL = 0.15 g/mL

9. C
8 mL × 1.07 = 8.56 g = 8560 mg

10. A
978 g ÷ 1000 mL = 0.978 g/mL

SECTION 3

INTRAVENOUS INFUSIONS AND FLOW RATES

QUESTIONS

1. A 1 liter bag of fluids must be infused to a patient over 6 hours. If the calibration of the IV tubing is 14 gtts/mL, how many drops per minute will there be? (Round answer to the nearest whole number.)

   a. 16 gtts/min
   b. 27 gtts/min
   c. 32 gtts/min
   d. 39 gtts/min

2. What is the infusion rate in mL/hour of a one liter bag of normal saline that is to be infused over 8 hours? (Round answer to the nearest whole number.)

   a. 48 mL/hr
   b. 76 mL/hr
   c. 125 mL/hr
   d. 137 mL/hr

3. A patient is to receive 9 mcg/min of digoxin. The concentration of the digoxin is 1 mg/500 mL of IV fluid. How many milliliters per hour will the patient receive?

   a. 270 mL/hr
   b. 310 mL/hr
   c. 330 mL/hr
   d. 380 mL/hr

4. A patient is to receive 100 milliliters per hour of an IV bag that is 1 liter. How many hours will the IV bag last?

   a. 7 hours
   b. 10 hours
   c. 12 hours
   d. 13 hours

5. An order is received for 1.25 liters of D5W, to be infused over 24 hours. If the IV administration set is calibrated to deliver 18 gtts/mL, how many drops per minute will there be? (Round answer to the nearest whole number.)

   a. 10 gtts/min
   b. 11 gtts/min
   c. 14 gtts/min
   d. 16 gtts/min

6. **An order is received for a heparin infusion with a concentration of 50,000 units/L. The preparation is to be infused at 1000 units/hr. What is the flow rate in mL/hr?**

 a. 10 mL/hr
 b. 20 mL/hr
 c. 45 mL/hr
 d. 50 mL/hr

7. **A patient is to receive 750 milliliters of ½ NS over 12 hours. Calculate how many grams of sodium chloride would be administered per hour.**

 a. 0.7 g/hr
 b. 0.12 g/hr
 c. 0.16 g/hr
 d. 0.28 g/hr

8. **If 250 milliliters of D50W is infused, how many grams of dextrose will the patient receive?**

 a. 75 g
 b. 100 g
 c. 125 g
 d. 250 g

9. **A pharmacist adds 20 milliliters of an electrolyte solution and 35 milliliters of a multivitamin solution to 1.5 liters of NS. If the infusion is to be administered over a period of 5 hours, what is the flow rate in mL/hr?**

 a. 200 mL/hr
 b. 220 mL/hr
 c. 272 mL/hr
 d. 311 mL/hr

10. **A medication order calls for an intravenous infusion of calcium chloride 10 grams to be added to 150 milliliters of NS. The pharmacy has available calcium chloride 3 mEq/mL. How many milliliters of calcium chloride must be used to prepare the admixture? (M.W. of $CaCl_2$ = 147)**

 a. 45.35 mL
 b. 51.75 mL
 c. 86.25 mL
 d. 93.45 mL

11. **A patient is to receive 4 mg/min of lidocaine. How many hours will a 250 milliliter bag of 5% lidocaine solution last?**

    a. 28 hours
    b. 36 hours
    c. 40 hours
    d. 52 hours

12. **A patient weighing 87 kilograms is to receive dopamine at a dose of 4 mcg/kg/min from a bag containing 100 milligrams of the medication in 500 milliliters of D5W. How many milliliters per hour should be infused to provide the desired dose of dopamine?**

    a. 73.4 mL/hr
    b. 82.9 mL/hr
    c. 104.4 mL/hr
    d. 110.8 mL/hr

The following information relates to questions 13 – 14.

A patient weighing 80 kilograms is to receive dobutamine 3 mcg/kg/min. The available solution contains 100 milligrams of the medication in 250 milliliters of D5W and the calibration of the IV tubing is 50 gtts/mL.

13. **How many milligrams of dobutamine will the patient receive per hour?**

    a. 9.8 mg/hr
    b. 11.2 mg/hr
    c. 13.6 mg/hr
    d. 14.4 mg/hr

14. **How many drops per minute will the patient receive? (Round answer to the nearest whole number.)**

    a. 30 gtts/min
    b. 42 gtts/min
    c. 45 gtts/min
    d. 57 gtts/min

15. **A 165 pound patient is to receive an intravenous infusion that contains 0.5 grams of nitroglycerin in 250 milliliters of D5W. An IV pump is programmed to deliver 3 mcg/kg/min. Calculate the flow rate in mL/hr.**

    a. 5.23 mL/hr
    b. 6.75 mL/hr
    c. 7.95 mL/hr
    d. 8.16 mL/hr

The following information relates to questions 16 – 18.

An intravenous infusion contains 400 milligrams of acyclovir in 100 milliliters of D5W. The infusion is to be administered over 60 minutes and the calibration of the IV tubing is set at 30 gtts/mL.

16. How many milligrams of acyclovir should be administered per minute?

    a. 5.48 mg/min
    b. 6.67 mg/min
    c. 6.94 mg/min
    d. 8.45 mg/min

17. How many milliliters of the acyclovir infusion should be administered per minute?

    a. 1.67 mL/min
    b. 2.18 mL/min
    c. 3.32 mL/min
    d. 4.57 mL/min

18. How many drops per minute should be infused? (Round answer to the nearest whole number.)

    a. 29 gtts/min
    b. 37 gtts/min
    c. 44 gtts/min
    d. 50 gtts/min

The following information relates to questions 19 – 21.

A hospital pharmacy receives an order for 50 milligrams of isoproterenol in 250 milliliters of D5W. A patient is to receive an initial infusion dose of 2 mcg/min that can be increased as necessary to a maximum dose of 20 mcg/min. The calibration of the IV tubing set to be used is 20 gtts/mL.

19. Calculate the concentration of isoproterenol in the infusion solution in mcg/mL.

    a. 125 mcg/mL
    b. 180 mcg/mL
    c. 200 mcg/mL
    d. 250 mcg/mL

20. Calculate the initial infusion dose in mL/hr.

    a. 0.6 mL/hr
    b. 0.9 mL/hr
    c. 1.2 mL/hr
    d. 1.3 mL/hr

21. Calculate the maximum infusion dose in gtts/min.

    a. 2 gtts/min
    b. 5 gtts/min
    c. 10 gtts/min
    d. 12 gtts/min

22. If 750 milliliters of NS is infused, how many milligrams of sodium chloride will the patient receive?

    a. 2250 mg
    b. 5450 mg
    c. 5920 mg
    d. 6750 mg

23. An intravenous drip contains 3 grams of labetalol and is to be administered at a rate of 4 mg/min. Calculate the total time of the infusion in hours.

    a. 10.25 hours
    b. 12.5 hours
    c. 15.5 hours
    d. 16.5 hours

24. A patient received 100 milliliters of NS at an infusion rate of 20 gtts/min with an IV tubing set that was calibrated to deliver 50 gtts/mL. Calculate the total time of the infusion in minutes.

    a. 120 minutes
    b. 160 minutes
    c. 185 minutes
    d. 250 minutes

25. A pharmacist adds 12 units of insulin to 750 milliliters of D5W. The infusion is to be administered intravenously over 8 hours. How many units of insulin would be administered in a 20 minute period?

    a. 0.3 units
    b. 0.5 units
    c. 0.8 units
    d. 1 unit

ANSWER KEY

1. D

$$\frac{1 \text{ L}}{6 \text{ hr}} \times \frac{1000 \text{ mL}}{1 \text{ L}} \times \frac{1 \text{ hr}}{60 \text{ min}} \times \frac{14 \text{ gtts}}{1 \text{ mL}} = 38.8 \text{ gtts/min} = 39 \text{ gtts/min}$$

2. C

$$\frac{1 \text{ L}}{8 \text{ hr}} \times \frac{1000 \text{ mL}}{1 \text{ L}} = 125 \text{ mL/hr}$$

3. A

$$\frac{9 \text{ mcg}}{1 \text{ min}} \times \frac{1 \text{ mg}}{1000 \text{ mcg}} \times \frac{500 \text{ mL}}{1 \text{ mg}} \times \frac{60 \text{ min}}{1 \text{ hr}} = 270 \text{ mL/hr}$$

4. B

1000 mL × 1 hr/100 mL = 10 hours

5. D

$$\frac{1.25 \text{ L}}{24 \text{ hr}} \times \frac{1000 \text{ mL}}{1 \text{ L}} \times \frac{24 \text{ hr}}{1440 \text{ min}} \times \frac{18 \text{ gtts}}{1 \text{ mL}} = 15.6 \text{ gtts/min} = 16 \text{ gtts/min}$$

6. B

$$\frac{1 \text{ L}}{50,000 \text{ units}} \times \frac{1000 \text{ mL}}{1 \text{ L}} \times \frac{1000 \text{ units}}{1 \text{ hr}} = 20 \text{ mL/hr}$$

7. D

$$\frac{0.45 \text{ g}}{100 \text{ mL}} \times \frac{750 \text{ mL}}{12 \text{ hr}} = 0.28 \text{ g/hr}$$

8. C

Step 1: $\dfrac{50 \text{ g}}{100 \text{ mL}} = \dfrac{x \text{ g}}{250 \text{ mL}}$

Step 2: $100x = 12{,}500$

Step 3: $x = 125$ g

9. D

Step 1: 20 mL + 35 mL + 1500 mL = 1555 mL
Step 2: 1555 mL ÷ 5 hr = 311 mL/hr

10. A

Step 1: Convert the concentration of the calcium chloride available to g/mL.

$$\frac{3 \text{ mEq}}{1 \text{ mL}} \times \frac{147 \text{ mg}}{1 \text{ mmol}} \times \frac{1 \text{ mmol}}{2 \text{ mEq}} \times \frac{1 \text{ g}}{1000 \text{ mg}} = 0.2205 \text{ g/mL}$$

Step 2: Calculate how many milliliters of calcium chloride are required to prepare the admixture.

a. $\dfrac{0.2205 \text{ g}}{1 \text{ mL}} = \dfrac{10 \text{ g}}{x \text{ mL}}$

b. $0.2205x = 10$

c. $x = 45.35$ mL

11. D

$250 \text{ mL} \times \dfrac{5 \text{ g}}{100 \text{ mL}} \times \dfrac{1000 \text{ mg}}{1 \text{ g}} \times \dfrac{1 \text{ min}}{4 \text{ mg}} \times \dfrac{1 \text{ hr}}{60 \text{ min}} = 52 \text{ hours}$

12. C

Step 1: Calculate the amount of dopamine needed per minute.
4 mcg/kg/min × 87 kg = 348 mcg/min

Step 2: Calculate how many milliliters per hour should be infused.

$\dfrac{500 \text{ mL}}{100 \text{ mg}} \times \dfrac{1 \text{ mg}}{1000 \text{ mcg}} \times \dfrac{348 \text{ mcg}}{1 \text{ min}} \times \dfrac{60 \text{ min}}{1 \text{ hr}} = 104.4 \text{ mL/hr}$

13. D

$80 \text{ kg} \times \dfrac{3 \text{ mcg}}{\text{kg/min}} \times \dfrac{1 \text{ mg}}{1000 \text{ mcg}} \times \dfrac{60 \text{ min}}{1 \text{ hr}} = 14.4 \text{ mg/hr}$

14. A

$\dfrac{14.4 \text{ mg}}{60 \text{ min}} \times \dfrac{250 \text{ mL}}{100 \text{ mg}} \times \dfrac{50 \text{ gtts}}{1 \text{ mL}} = 30 \text{ gtts/min}$

15. B

$165 \text{ lb} \times \dfrac{1 \text{ kg}}{2.2 \text{ lb}} \times \dfrac{3 \text{ mcg}}{\text{kg/min}} \times \dfrac{250 \text{ mL}}{0.5 \text{ g}} \times \dfrac{1 \text{ mg}}{1000 \text{ mcg}} \times \dfrac{1 \text{ g}}{1000 \text{ mg}} \times \dfrac{60 \text{ min}}{1 \text{ hr}} = 6.75 \text{ mL/hr}$

16. B

400 mg/60 min = 6.67 mg/min

17. A

$\dfrac{6.67 \text{ mg}}{1 \text{ min}} \times \dfrac{100 \text{ mL}}{400 \text{ mg}} = 1.67 \text{ mL/min}$

18. D

$\dfrac{1.67 \text{ mL}}{1 \text{ min}} \times \dfrac{30 \text{ gtts}}{1 \text{ mL}} = 50.1 \text{ gtts/min} = 50 \text{ gtts/min}$

19. C

$\dfrac{50 \text{ mg}}{250 \text{ mL}} \times \dfrac{1000 \text{ mcg}}{1 \text{ mg}} = 200 \text{ mcg/mL}$

20. A

$$\frac{1\ mL}{200\ mcg} \times \frac{2\ mcg}{1\ min} \times \frac{60\ min}{1\ hr} = 0.6\ mL/hr$$

21. A

$$\frac{1\ mL}{200\ mcg} \times \frac{20\ mcg}{1\ min} \times \frac{20\ gtts}{1\ mL} = 2\ gtts/min$$

22. D

Step 1: $\dfrac{0.9\ g}{100\ mL} = \dfrac{x\ g}{750\ mL}$

Step 2: $100x = 675$

Step 3: $x = 6.75\ g \times 1000 = 6750\ mg$

23. B

$$3\ g \times \frac{1000\ mg}{1\ g} \times \frac{1\ min}{4\ mg} \times \frac{1\ hr}{60\ min} = 12.5\ hours$$

24. D

$$100\ mL \times \frac{50\ gtts}{1\ mL} \times \frac{1\ min}{20\ gtts} = 250\ minutes$$

25. B

$$\frac{12\ units}{8\ hr} \times \frac{1\ hr}{60\ min} \times 20\ min = 0.5\ units$$

SECTION 4

REDUCING AND ENLARGING FORMULAS

QUESTIONS

The following information relates to questions 1 – 4.

Rx:
Coal tar	2 parts
Zinc oxide	6 parts
Glycerin	3 parts
White petrolatum	8 parts

1. **How many grams of coal tar are needed to make 500 grams of the above prescription?**

   a. 52.6 g
   b. 58.3 g
   c. 64.5 g
   d. 71.4 g

2. **How many grams of zinc oxide are needed to make 500 grams of the above prescription?**

   a. 129.8 g
   b. 133.5 g
   c. 138.2 g
   d. 157.9 g

3. **How many grams of glycerin are needed to make 500 grams of the above prescription?**

   a. 49.8 g
   b. 63.2 g
   c. 78.9 g
   d. 84.7 g

4. **How many grams of white petrolatum are needed to make 500 grams of the above prescription?**

   a. 210.5 g
   b. 273.8 g
   c. 294.7 g
   d. 301.6 g

5. The formula to prepare 450 milliliters of a lotion contains 8 grams of hydrocortisone. How many milligrams of hydrocortisone are needed to prepare 120 milliliters of the lotion?

   a. 1614.7 mg
   b. 1986.9 mg
   c. 2133.3 mg
   d. 2376.2 mg

The following formula for 25 furosemide capsules relates to questions 6 – 8.

Furosemide	250 mg
Silica gel	4 g
Lactose	5 g

6. Calculate how many grams of furosemide are needed to prepare 60 capsules.

   a. 0.4 g
   b. 0.6 g
   c. 0.9 g
   d. 1.3 g

7. Calculate how many grams of silica gel are needed to prepare 60 capsules.

   a. 4.5 g
   b. 6.2 g
   c. 7.1 g
   d. 9.6 g

8. Calculate how many grams of lactose are needed to prepare 60 capsules.

   a. 4 g
   b. 7 g
   c. 12 g
   d. 14 g

9. The formula to prepare one liter of a sodium chloride solution calls for 150 grams of sodium chloride. How many grams of sodium chloride are needed to prepare one pint of the solution?

   a. 70.95 g
   b. 82.37 g
   c. 114.95 g
   d. 126.54 g

The following formula relates to questions 10 – 13.

Bacitracin 500 units/gram ointment	2 parts
Hydrocortisone 2.5% ointment	1 part
Nystatin 100,000 units/gram ointment	4 parts
Zinc oxide 40% ointment	5 parts

10. **How many grams of bacitracin 500 units/gram ointment are needed to prepare 80 grams of the above formula?**

    a. 8.83 g
    b. 9.43 g
    c. 12.67 g
    d. 13.33 g

11. **How many grams of hydrocortisone 2.5% ointment are needed to prepare 80 grams of the above formula?**

    a. 4.91 g
    b. 6.67 g
    c. 9.24 g
    d. 10.27 g

12. **How many grams of nystatin 100,000 units/gram ointment are needed to prepare 80 grams of the above formula?**

    a. 26.67 g
    b. 32.86 g
    c. 34.92 g
    d. 38.96 g

13. **How many grams of zinc oxide 40% ointment are needed to prepare 80 grams of the above formula?**

    a. 28.95 g
    b. 30.76 g
    c. 33.33 g
    d. 43.32 g

The following formula relates to questions 14 – 15.

Oxymetazoline 0.05% solution   30 mL
Sodium chloride 0.9% solution for injection 45 mL

14. Calculate how many milliliters of oxymetazoline 0.05% solution are needed to prepare 90 milliliters of the above formula.

    a. 24 mL
    b. 29 mL
    c. 31 mL
    d. 36 mL

15. Calculate how many milliliters of sodium chloride 0.9% solution for injection are needed to prepare 90 milliliters of the above formula.

    a. 42 mL
    b. 47 mL
    c. 54 mL
    d. 60 mL

ANSWER KEY

1. A

Step 1: Total parts = 2 + 6 + 3 + 8 = 19

Step 2: $\dfrac{500 \text{ g}}{19 \text{ parts}} = \dfrac{x \text{ g}}{2 \text{ parts}}$

Step 3: $19x = 1000$

Step 4: $x = 52.6$ g

2. D

Step 1: Total parts = 2 + 6 + 3 + 8 = 19

Step 2: $\dfrac{500 \text{ g}}{19 \text{ parts}} = \dfrac{x \text{ g}}{6 \text{ parts}}$

Step 3: $19x = 3000$

Step 4: $x = 157.9$ g

3. C

Step 1: Total parts = 2 + 6 + 3 + 8 = 19

Step 2: $\dfrac{500 \text{ g}}{19 \text{ parts}} = \dfrac{x \text{ g}}{3 \text{ parts}}$

Step 3: $19x = 1500$

Step 4: $x = 78.9$ g

4. A

Step 1: Total parts = 2 + 6 + 3 + 8 = 19

Step 2: $\dfrac{500 \text{ g}}{19 \text{ parts}} = \dfrac{x \text{ g}}{8 \text{ parts}}$

Step 3: $19x = 4000$

Step 4: $x = 210.5$ g

5. C

Step 1: $\dfrac{8 \text{ g}}{450 \text{ mL}} = \dfrac{x \text{ g}}{120 \text{ mL}}$

Step 2: $450x = 960$

Step 3: $x = 2.1333$ g × 1000 = 2133.3 mg

6. B

Step 1: $\dfrac{250 \text{ mg}}{25 \text{ caps}} = \dfrac{x \text{ mg}}{60 \text{ caps}}$

Step 2: $25x = 15{,}000$

Step 3: $x = 600$ mg ÷ 1000 = 0.6 g

7. D

Step 1: $\dfrac{4 \text{ g}}{25 \text{ caps}} = \dfrac{x \text{ g}}{60 \text{ caps}}$

Step 2: $25x = 240$

Step 3: $x = 9.6 \text{ g}$

8. C

Step 1: $\dfrac{5 \text{ g}}{25 \text{ caps}} = \dfrac{x \text{ g}}{60 \text{ caps}}$

Step 2: $25x = 300$

Step 3: $x = 12 \text{ g}$

9. A

Step 1: $\dfrac{150 \text{ g}}{1000 \text{ mL}} = \dfrac{x \text{ g}}{473 \text{ mL}}$

Step 2: $1000x = 70{,}950$

Step 3: $x = 70.95 \text{ g}$

10. D

Step 1: Total parts = 2 + 1 + 4 + 5 = 12 parts

Step 2: $\dfrac{80 \text{ g}}{12 \text{ parts}} = \dfrac{x \text{ g}}{2 \text{ parts}}$

Step 3: $12x = 160$

Step 4: $x = 13.33 \text{ g}$

11. B

Step 1: Total parts = 2 + 1 + 4 + 5 = 12 parts

Step 2: $\dfrac{80 \text{ g}}{12 \text{ parts}} = \dfrac{x \text{ g}}{1 \text{ part}}$

Step 3: $12x = 80$

Step 4: $x = 6.67 \text{ g}$

12. A

Step 1: Total parts = 2 + 1 + 4 + 5 = 12 parts

Step 2: $\dfrac{80 \text{ g}}{12 \text{ parts}} = \dfrac{x \text{ g}}{4 \text{ parts}}$

Step 3: $12x = 320$

Step 4: $x = 26.67 \text{ g}$

13. C

Step 1: Total parts = 2 + 1 + 4 + 5 = 12 parts

Step 2: $\dfrac{80 \text{ g}}{12 \text{ parts}} = \dfrac{x \text{ g}}{5 \text{ parts}}$

Step 3: $12x = 400$

Step 4: $x = 33.33$ g

14. D

Step 1: Total volume of formula = 30 mL + 45 mL = 75 mL

Step 2: $\dfrac{30 \text{ mL}}{75 \text{ mL}} = \dfrac{x \text{ mL}}{90 \text{ mL}}$

Step 3: $75x = 2700$

Step 4: $x = 36$ mL

15. C

Step 1: Total volume of formula = 30 mL + 45 mL = 75 mL

Step 2: $\dfrac{45 \text{ mL}}{75 \text{ mL}} = \dfrac{x \text{ mL}}{90 \text{ mL}}$

Step 3: $75x = 4050$

Step 4: $x = 54$ mL

SECTION 5

ELECTROLYTE SOLUTIONS

QUESTIONS

1. A solution contains 20 mg% concentration of chloride ions. Convert the concentration to mEq/L. (M.W. of Cl = 35.5)

    a. 0.56 mEq/L
    b. 2.82 mEq/L
    c. 3.26 mEq/L
    d. 5.63 mEq/L

2. Calculate the osmolarity of a solution containing 7.5% dextrose and 0.9% sodium chloride. (M.W. of $C_6H_{14}O_7$ = 180; M.W. of NaCl = 58.4)

    a. 335.78 mOsm/L
    b. 514.57 mOsm/L
    c. 724.89 mOsm/L
    d. 872.24 mOsm/L

3. How many millimoles of potassium chloride are present in 115 grams of the substance? (M.W. of KCl = 74.5)

    a. 648 mmol
    b. 832 mmol
    c. 1544 mmol
    d. 1982 mmol

4. A patient is to receive 5 milliequivalents of sodium per day. The pharmacy has available a 180 milliliter bottle of a 15% sodium chloride solution. How many doses are in the bottle? (M.W. of NaCl = 58.4; M.W. of Na = 23; M.W. of Cl = 35.4)

    a. 92 doses
    b. 105 doses
    c. 113 doses
    d. 124 doses

5. Convert 60 mEq/5 mL sodium chloride to mOsm/L. (M.W. of NaCl = 58.4)

    a. 6000 mOsm/L
    b. 19,000 mOsm/L
    c. 24,000 mOsm/L
    d. 32,000 mOsm/L

6. A medication order calls for an intravenous infusion of calcium chloride 20 grams to be added to 250 milliliters of NS. The pharmacy has available calcium chloride 4 mEq/mL. How many milliliters of calcium chloride must be used to prepare the admixture? (M.W. of $CaCl_2$ = 147)

    a. 47 mL
    b. 68 mL
    c. 96 mL
    d. 115 mL

7. Calculate how many milliequivalents of calcium are in 200 milliliters of 4.5% calcium chloride solution. (M.W. of $CaCl_2$ = 147)

    a. 52.92 mEq
    b. 76.53 mEq
    c. 103.88 mEq
    d. 122.45 mEq

8. A solution contains 12% glucose. Convert the concentration to mOsm/L. (M.W. of $C_6H_{12}O_6$ = 180)

    a. 337.73 mOsm/L
    b. 512.63 mOsm/L
    c. 547.92 mOsm/L
    d. 666.67 mOsm/L

9. Calculate how many grams of magnesium sulfate would be needed to prepare 180 milliliters of a solution containing 40 milliosmoles of magnesium sulfate. (M.W. of $MgSO_4$ = 120.4)

    a. 2.12 g
    b. 2.41 g
    c. 3.75 g
    d. 4.82 g

10. Convert 40 mEq/10 mL ammonium chloride to mmol/L. (M.W. of NH_4Cl = 53.5)

    a. 1600 mmol/L
    b. 2900 mmol/L
    c. 4000 mmol/L
    d. 4200 mmol/L

11. **How many millimoles of sodium chloride are present in 200 milliliters of a 15% w/v sodium chloride solution? (M.W. of NaCl = 58.4)**

   a. 364.1 mmol
   b. 513.7 mmol
   c. 591.8 mmol
   d. 662.8 mmol

12. **Calculate how many milliequivalents of sodium are present in an admixture that is prepared by adding a 10 milliliter vial of sodium chloride (2.5 mEq/mL) to 500 milliliters of ½ NS. (M.W. of NaCl = 58.4; M.W. of Na = 23; M.W. of Cl = 35.4)**

   a. 41.12 mEq
   b. 63.53 mEq
   c. 82.61 mEq
   d. 97.82 mEq

13. **Calculate how many milliosmoles of chloride are in 30 milliliters of 25% magnesium chloride solution. (M.W. of $MgCl_2$ = 95)**

   a. 85.93 mOsm
   b. 157.89 mOsm
   c. 182.36 mOsm
   d. 236.8 mOsm

14. **Calculate the concentration in milligrams per milliliter of a solution containing 8 mEq of calcium chloride per milliliter. (M.W. of $CaCl_2$ = 147)**

   a. 588 mg/mL
   b. 752 mg/mL
   c. 947 mg/mL
   d. 1176 mg/mL

15. **Convert 20 mEq/10 mL aluminum hydroxide to mg/L. (M.W. of $AlOH_3$ = 78)**

   a. 52,000 mg/L
   b. 83,800 mg/L
   c. 156,000 mg/L
   d. 227,900 mg/L

ANSWER KEY

1. D

$$\frac{20\text{ mg}}{100\text{ mL}} \times \frac{1000\text{ mL}}{1\text{ L}} \times \frac{1\text{ mEq}}{35.5\text{ mg}} = 5.63\text{ mEq/L}$$

2. C

Step 1: Calculate the osmolarity of 7.5% dextrose.

$$\frac{7.5\text{ g}}{100\text{ mL}} \times \frac{1000\text{ mg}}{1\text{ g}} \times \frac{1000\text{ mL}}{1\text{ L}} \times \frac{1\text{ mOsm}}{180\text{ mg}} = 416.67\text{ mOsm/L}$$

Step 2: Calculate the osmolarity of 0.9% sodium chloride.

$$\frac{0.9\text{ g}}{100\text{ mL}} \times \frac{1000\text{ mg}}{1\text{ g}} \times \frac{1000\text{ mL}}{1\text{ L}} \times \frac{2\text{ mOsm}}{58.4\text{ mg}} = 308.22\text{ mOsm/L}$$

Step 3: Calculate the sum of step 1 and step 2.
416.67 mOsm/L + 308.22 mOsm/L = 724.89 mOsm/L

3. C

Step 1: $\dfrac{74.5\text{ g}}{1\text{ mole}} = \dfrac{115\text{ g}}{x\text{ mole}}$

Step 2: $74.5x = 115$

Step 3: $x = 1.544$ moles $\times 1000 = 1544$ mmol

4. A

Step 1: Calculate how many milliequivalents of sodium are in the stock bottle.

$$180\text{ mL} \times \frac{15\text{ g NaCl}}{100\text{ mL}} \times \frac{1000\text{ mg NaCl}}{1\text{ g NaCl}} \times \frac{1\text{ mmol NaCl}}{58.4\text{ mg NaCl}} \times \frac{1\text{ mEq NaCl}}{1\text{ mmol NaCl}} \times \frac{1\text{ mEq Na}}{1\text{ mEq NaCl}}$$
$$= 462.3\text{ mEq}$$

Step 2: Calculate how many doses are in the bottle.
462.3 mEq × 1 dose/5 mEq = 92 doses

5. C

$$\frac{60\text{ mEq}}{5\text{ mL}} \times \frac{1\text{ mmol}}{1\text{ mEq}} \times \frac{2\text{ mOsm}}{1\text{ mmol}} \times \frac{1000\text{ mL}}{1\text{ L}} = 24{,}000\text{ mOsm/L}$$

6. B

Step 1: Convert the concentration of the calcium chloride available to g/mL.

$$\frac{4\text{ mEq}}{1\text{ mL}} \times \frac{147\text{ mg}}{1\text{ mmol}} \times \frac{1\text{ mmol}}{2\text{ mEq}} \times \frac{1\text{ g}}{1000\text{ mg}} = 0.294\text{ g/mL}$$

Step 2: Calculate how many milliliters of calcium chloride are required to prepare the admixture.

a. $\dfrac{0.294\text{ g}}{1\text{ mL}} = \dfrac{20\text{ g}}{x\text{ mL}}$

b. $0.294x = 20$

c. $x = 68\text{ mL}$

7. D

$$200 \text{ mL} \times \frac{4.5 \text{ g CaCl}_2}{100 \text{ mL}} \times \frac{1000 \text{ mg CaCl}_2}{1 \text{ g CaCl}_2} \times \frac{1 \text{ mmol CaCl}_2}{147 \text{ mg CaCl}_2} \times \frac{2 \text{ mEq CaCl}_2}{1 \text{ mmol CaCl}_2} \times \frac{1 \text{ mEq Ca}}{1 \text{ mEq CaCl}_2}$$
$$= 122.45 \text{ mEq Ca}$$

8. D

$$\frac{12 \text{ g}}{100 \text{ mL}} \times \frac{1000 \text{ mg}}{1 \text{ g}} \times \frac{1000 \text{ mL}}{1 \text{ L}} \times \frac{1 \text{ mOsm}}{180 \text{ mg}} = 666.67 \text{ mOsm/L}$$

9. B

$$40 \text{ mOsm} \times \frac{120.4 \text{ mg}}{2 \text{ mOsm}} \times \frac{1 \text{ g}}{1000 \text{ mg}} = 2.41 \text{ g}$$

10. C

$$\frac{40 \text{ mEq}}{10 \text{ mL}} \times \frac{1 \text{ mmol}}{1 \text{ mEq}} \times \frac{1000 \text{ mL}}{1 \text{ L}} = 4000 \text{ mmol/L}$$

11. B

Step 1: Calculate the amount of sodium chloride in 200 milliliters of a 15% w/v sodium chloride solution.

a. $\dfrac{15 \text{ g}}{100 \text{ mL}} = \dfrac{x \text{ g}}{200 \text{ mL}}$

b. $100x = 3000$

c. $x = 30 \text{ g}$

Step 2: Calculate how many moles of sodium chloride are in 200 milliliters of a 15% w/v sodium chloride solution.

a. $\dfrac{58.4 \text{ g}}{1 \text{ mole}} = \dfrac{30 \text{ g}}{x \text{ mole}}$

b. $58.4x = 30$

c. $x = 0.5137 \text{ mole} \times 1000 = 513.7 \text{ mmol}$

12. B

Step 1: Calculate how many milliequivalents of sodium are present in the vial of sodium chloride.

$$10 \text{ mL} \times \frac{2.5 \text{ mEq NaCl}}{1 \text{ mL}} \times \frac{1 \text{ mEq NaCl}}{1 \text{ mmol NaCl}} \times \frac{1 \text{ mEq Na}}{1 \text{ mEq NaCl}} = 25 \text{ mEq Na}$$

Step 2: Calculate how many milliequivalents of sodium are present in 500 milliliters of ½ NS.

$$500 \text{ mL} \times \frac{0.45 \text{ g NaCl}}{100 \text{ mL}} \times \frac{1000 \text{ mg}}{1 \text{ g}} \times \frac{1 \text{ mmol NaCl}}{58.4 \text{ mg NaCl}} \times \frac{1 \text{ mEq NaCl}}{1 \text{ mmol NaCl}} \times \frac{1 \text{ mEq Na}}{1 \text{ mEq NaCl}}$$
$$= 38.53 \text{ mEq Na}$$

Step 3: Calculate the sum of step 1 and step 2.
25 mEq + 38.53 mEq = 63.53 mEq

13. B

$$30 \text{ mL} \times \frac{25 \text{ g MgCl}_2}{100 \text{ mL}} \times \frac{1000 \text{ mg MgCl}_2}{1 \text{ g MgCl}_2} \times \frac{1 \text{ mmol MgCl}_2}{95 \text{ mg MgCl}_2} \times \frac{2 \text{ mOsm Cl}}{1 \text{ mmol MgCl}_2}$$
$$= 157.89 \text{ mOsm Cl}$$

14. A

$$\frac{8 \text{ mEq}}{1 \text{ mL}} \times \frac{1 \text{ mmol}}{2 \text{ mEq}} \times \frac{147 \text{ mg}}{1 \text{ mmol}} = 588 \text{ mg/mL}$$

15. A

$$\frac{20 \text{ mEq}}{10 \text{ mL}} \times \frac{78 \text{ mg}}{3 \text{ mEq}} \times \frac{1000 \text{ mL}}{1 \text{ L}} = 52,000 \text{ mg/L}$$

SECTION 6

ISOTONIC AND BUFFER SOLUTIONS

QUESTIONS

1. What is the pH of a buffer solution prepared with 0.05 M ammonia (pK$_b$ = 4.74) and 0.005 M ammonium chloride?

   a. 9.53
   b. 10.26
   c. 11.16
   d. 11.84

2. Calculate how many grams of sodium chloride are needed to compound the following prescription. (The E-value for pilocarpine nitrate is 0.23.)

   Rx:
   Pilocarpine nitrate   0.4 g
   Sodium chloride   qs
   Purified water   ad 30 mL
   Make isotonic solution
   Sig: i gtt od tid

   a. 0.092 g
   b. 0.106 g
   c. 0.178 g
   d. 0.194 g

3. Calculate the E value for potassium nitrate, which dissociates into 2 particles. (M.W. = 101)

   a. 0.29
   b. 0.47
   c. 0.58
   d. 0.84

4. Calculate how many grams of boric acid are needed to compound the following prescription. (The E value for cromolyn sodium is 0.14; the E value for boric acid is 0.52.)

   Rx:
   Cromolyn sodium   0.5 g
   Boric acid   qs
   Purified water   ad 60 mL
   Make isotonic solution
   Sig: i gtt od bid

   a. 0.372 g
   b. 0.491 g
   c. 0.658 g
   d. 0.904 g

5. How many milligrams of sodium chloride are needed to prepare 100 milliliters of a 1% solution of naphazoline hydrochloride that is isotonic? (The D value of naphazoline hydrochloride 1% is 0.16.)

a. 623 mg
b. 658 mg
c. 763 mg
d. 810 mg

6. The dissociation constant of lactic acid is 1.38×10^{-4} at 25°C. Calculate its pKa value.

a. 2.65
b. 3.11
c. 3.86
d. 4.27

7. Calculate the E value for zinc chloride, which dissociates into 3 particles. (M.W. = 136)

a. 0.29
b. 0.43
c. 0.62
d. 0.81

8. What is the pH of a buffer solution prepared with 0.65 M sodium acetate and 0.065 M acetic acid (pK$_a$ = 4.76)?

a. 4.76
b. 5.28
c. 5.76
d. 6.17

9. Calcium chloride (CaCl$_2$) is a 3-ion electrolyte that dissociates 60% in a certain concentration. Calculate its dissociation (*i*) factor.

a. 2.2
b. 2.6
c. 3.2
d. 3.8

10. **Calculate the change in pH after adding 0.05 mol of sodium hydroxide to one liter of a buffer solution containing 0.1 M concentrations each of sodium acetate and acetic acid (pK$_a$ = 4.76).**

    a. 0.21
    b. 0.24
    c. 0.39
    d. 0.48

ANSWER KEY

1. B

$$pH = 14 - 4.74 + \log \frac{0.05}{0.005} = 10.26$$

2. C

Step 1: Calculate the amount of sodium chloride represented from pilocarpine nitrate.
0.4 g × 0.23 = 0.092 g

Step 2: Calculate the amount of sodium chloride that will make the solution isotonic.

a. $\dfrac{0.9 \text{ g}}{100 \text{ mL}} = \dfrac{x \text{ g}}{30 \text{ mL}}$

b. $100x = 27$

c. $x = 0.27$ g

Step 3: Subtract step 1 from step 2.
0.27 g – 0.092 g = 0.178 g of sodium chloride is needed to make an isotonic solution.

3. C

$$E = \frac{58.5 \times 1.8}{101 \times 1.8} = 0.58$$

4. D

Step 1: Calculate the amount of sodium chloride represented from cromolyn sodium.
0.5 g × 0.14 = 0.07 g

Step 2: Calculate the amount of sodium chloride that will make a 60 mL solution isotonic.

a. $\dfrac{0.9 \text{ g}}{100 \text{ mL}} = \dfrac{x \text{ g}}{60 \text{ mL}}$

b. $100x = 54$

c. $x = 0.54$ g

Step 3: Subtract step 1 from step 2 to calculate the amount of sodium chloride that will make the compounded solution isotonic.
0.54 g – 0.07 g = 0.47 g

Step 4: Calculate the amount of boric acid required to make the solution isotonic.
0.47 g ÷ 0.52 = 0.904 g

5. A

Step 1: Calculate how much the freezing point needs to be lowered by to be isotonic.
0.52°C – 0.16°C = 0.36°C

Step 2: Calculate the amount (percent strength) of sodium chloride that is required to lower the freezing point.

a. $\dfrac{0.9\% \text{ NaCl}}{0.52°C} = \dfrac{x\% \text{ NaCl}}{0.36°C}$

b. $0.52x = 0.324$

c. $x = 0.623\%$

Step 3: Convert the percent strength of sodium chloride that is required to milligrams.

$\dfrac{0.623 \text{ g}}{100 \text{ mL}} \times \dfrac{1000 \text{ mg}}{1 \text{ g}} \times 100 \text{ mL} = 623 \text{ mg}$

6. C

$pK_a = -\log (1.38 \times 10^{-4}) = 3.86$

7. C

$E = \dfrac{58.5 \times 2.6}{136 \times 1.8} = 0.62$

8. C

$pH = 4.76 + \log \dfrac{0.65}{0.065} = 5.76$

9. A

Each 100 molecules will yield:

    60 calcium ions
   120 chloride ions
 + 40 undissociated particles
  220 particles total

Thus, the dissociation (i) factor = 220/100 = 2.2

10. D

Step 1: Calculate the pH of the buffer solution.

$pH = 4.76 + \log \dfrac{0.1}{0.1} = 4.76$

Step 2: Calculate the pH of the solution after the addition of the sodium hydroxide.

$pH = 4.76 + \log \dfrac{0.1 + 0.05}{0.1 - 0.05} = 5.24$

Step 3: Subtract step 1 from step 2 to calculate the change in pH of the solution after the addition of the sodium hydroxide.

$5.24 - 4.76 = 0.48$

SECTION 7

DILUTIONS AND CONCENTRATIONS

QUESTIONS

1. **Calculate how many grams of 1.5% ointment can be made from 24 grams of salicylic acid.**

   a. 625 g
   b. 1150 g
   c. 1600 g
   d. 1360 g

2. **How many milliliters of a 12% w/v stock solution are needed to prepare 150 milliliters of a solution that has a concentration of 20 mg/mL of the active ingredient?**

   a. 10 mL
   b. 16 mL
   c. 25 mL
   d. 34 mL

3. **A prescription calls for 250 milliliters of 0.85% ranitidine solution. How many liters of 0.25% ranitidine solution will be needed to prepare the prescription?**

   a. 0.85 L
   b. 1.5 L
   c. 2.15 L
   d. 2.5 L

4. **How many milliliters each of alcohol 91% and alcohol 70% should be mixed to prepare one liter of alcohol 85% solution?**

   a. 188.3 mL of alcohol 70% and 811.7 mL of alcohol 91%
   b. 217.5 mL of alcohol 70% and 782.5 mL of alcohol 91%
   c. 251.4 mL of alcohol 70% and 748.6 mL of alcohol 91%
   d. 285.7 mL of alcohol 70% and 714.3 mL of alcohol 91%

5. **A prescription calls for 60 milliliters of 0.15% prednisolone solution. How many milliliters of 0.5% prednisolone solution will be needed to prepare the prescription?**

   a. 10 mL
   b. 18 mL
   c. 30 mL
   d. 36 mL

6. How many grams of white petrolatum should be added to 75 grams of a 40% urea ointment to make a 15% ointment?

    a. 125 g
    b. 152 g
    c. 194 g
    d. 210 g

7. Calculate the specific gravity of a mixture of 10 milliliters of peppermint oil (SG = 0.90), 30 milliliters of propylene glycol (SG = 1.03), and 70 milliliters of glycerin (SG = 1.25).

    a. 0.92
    b. 0.98
    c. 1.07
    d. 1.16

8. How many milliliters of 20% sucrose can be made from one pint of 70% sucrose?

    a. 1435.7 mL
    b. 1655.5 mL
    c. 1926.1 mL
    d. 2015.4 mL

9. Lidocaine injection is available in a 5 milliliter vial that contains 20 mg/mL. If the injection is diluted by adding the contents of one vial to a 500 milliliter bag of NS, calculate the percent concentration of lidocaine in the bag of NS.

    a. 0.02%
    b. 0.06%
    c. 0.21%
    d. 0.37%

10. If one pint of a 25% w/v solution is diluted to one liter, calculate the percent strength of the diluted solution.

    a. 11.8%
    b. 12.5%
    c. 14.7%
    d. 15.1%

11. **Calculate how many milliliters of chlorhexidine gluconate are required to pre-pare the following prescription. The source of chlorhexidine gluconate to be used is 4% w/w solution and its specific gravity is 1.06.**

Rx:
Chlorhexidine gluconate 2.5% w/v solution
Disp. 480 mL
Sig: Wash affected areas bid

   a. 112 mL
   b. 249 mL
   c. 283 mL
   d. 318 mL

12. **If one pint of 16% lactic acid is diluted to two quarts with water, what is the ratio strength of the diluted solution?**

   a. 1:10
   b. 1:12
   c. 1:18
   d. 1:25

13. **Calculate how many milliliters of a 4% stock solution of potassium hydroxide should be used to compound the following prescription.**

Rx:
Potassium hydroxide solution 1:5000
Dispense 120 mL
Sig: use as directed

   a. 0.2 mL
   b. 0.6 mL
   c. 1.2 mL
   d. 1.8 mL

14. **How many milliliters of water must be added to 120 milliliters of a 15% ben-zalkonium chloride solution to prepare a 2.5% solution of benzalkonium chlo-ride?**

   a. 330 mL
   b. 580 mL
   c. 600 mL
   d. 720 mL

15. How many grams each of hydrocortisone 2.5% ointment and white petrolatum should be mixed to prepare 240 grams of hydrocortisone 1.75% ointment?

    a. 127 g of hydrocortisone 2.5% ointment and 113 g of white petrolatum
    b. 168 g of hydrocortisone 2.5% ointment and 72 g of white petrolatum
    c. 190 g of hydrocortisone 2.5% ointment and 50 g of white petrolatum
    d. 202 g of hydrocortisone 2.5% ointment and 38 g of white petrolatum

16. How many milliliters of 85% w/w hydrochloric acid (SG = 1.37) should be used to prepare one gallon of 25% w/v acid?

    a. 516.1 mL
    b. 743.9 mL
    c. 812.6 mL
    d. 1037.8 mL

17. How many grams of 40% w/w zinc oxide can be made from one pound of 65% w/w zinc oxide?

    a. 279.38 g
    b. 458.26 g
    c. 639.14 g
    d. 737.75 g

18. If 60 grams of 2% mupirocin ointment are mixed with 15 grams of white petrolatum, calculate the final concentration of mupirocin in the mixture.

    a. 0.5%
    b. 0.9%
    c. 1.2%
    d. 1.6%

19. How many milliliters of 30% acetic acid stock solution are required to make 180 milliliters of 12% acetic acid solution?

    a. 30 mL
    b. 48 mL
    c. 72 mL
    d. 110 mL

20. **Calculate how many milliliters of a 2.5% w/v solution of menthol in alcohol should be used to obtain the amount of menthol required to prepare the following prescription.**

    Rx:
    Menthol
    Camphor   aa 0.75%
    Glycerin   15%
    70% isopropyl alcohol   qs 240 mL

    a. 18 mL
    b. 34 mL
    c. 51 mL
    d. 72 mL

21. **How many grams of epinephrine should be used to prepare 500 milliliters of a stock solution such that when 30 milliliters is diluted to 750 milliliters, the final solution will have a percent strength of 1% w/v?**

    a. 44 g
    b. 72 g
    c. 96 g
    d. 125 g

22. **Calculate the percent strength (w/w) of fluocinolone in a cream prepared by mixing 30 grams of 0.01% cream, 70 grams of 0.025% cream, and 20 grams of 0.035% cream.**

    a. 0.018%
    b. 0.023%
    c. 0.036%
    d. 0.045%

23. **How many milliliters of a 1:80 w/v stock solution of sodium chloride should be used to prepare two liters of a 1:1000 w/v solution of sodium chloride?**

    a. 32 mL
    b. 160 mL
    c. 256 mL
    d. 315 mL

24. How many grams each of urea 10% cream and urea 40% cream should be mixed to prepare 180 grams of urea 30% cream?

a. 60 g of urea 10% cream and 120 g of urea 40% cream
b. 95 g of urea 10% cream and 85 g of urea 40% cream
c. 110 g of urea 0.10% cream and 70 g of urea 40% cream
d. 125 g of urea 10% cream and 55 g of urea 40% cream

25. How many milliliters of water must be added to 60 milliliters of 1.75% sodium chloride solution to make a 1:500 sodium chloride solution?

a. 415 mL
b. 465 mL
c. 525 mL
d. 600 mL

ANSWER KEY

1. C

Step 1: $\dfrac{1.5 \text{ g}}{100 \text{ g}} = \dfrac{24 \text{ g}}{x \text{ g}}$

Step 2: $1.5x = 2400$

Step 3: $x = 1600$ g

2. C

Step 1: Convert the desired final concentration of the active ingredient to a percent strength.

a. 20 mg/mL × 150 mL = 3000 mg ÷ 1000 = 3 g

b. $\dfrac{3 \text{ g}}{150 \text{ mL}} = \dfrac{x \text{ g}}{100 \text{ mL}}$

c. $150x = 300$

d. $x = 2$ g of active ingredient in 100 mL of solution, therefore the percent strength is 2%.

Step 2: Calculate how many milliliters of the stock solution are needed.

a. 12% × x mL = 2% × 150 mL

b. $12x = 300$

c. $x = 25$ mL

3. A

Step 1: 0.25% × x mL = 0.85% × 250 mL

Step 2: $0.25x = 212.5$

Step 3: $x = 850$ mL ÷ 1000 = 0.85 L

4. D

Percentage		Parts
91%		15 parts
	85%	
70%		6 parts
		21 total parts

Quantity of 70% alcohol: 1000 mL × 6/21 = 285.7 mL
Quantity of 91% alcohol: 1000 mL × 15/21 = 714.3 mL

5. B
Step 1: 0.5% × x mL = 0.15% × 60 mL
Step 2: $0.5x = 9$
Step 3: $x = 18$ mL

6. A
Step 1: 15% × (x + 75 g) = 40% × 75 g
Step 2: $15x + 1125 = 3000$
Step 3: $15x = 1875$
Step 4: $x = 125$ g

7. D
$$\frac{\sum[(0.90 \times 10 \text{ mL}) + (1.03 \times 30 \text{ mL}) + (1.25 \times 70 \text{ mL})]}{110 \text{ mL}} = 1.16$$

8. B
Step 1: 20% × x mL = 70% × 473 mL
Step 2: $20x = 33{,}110$
Step 3: $x = 1655.5$ mL

9. A
Step 1: Calculate the percent strength of lidocaine in the vial.
a. $\dfrac{0.02 \text{ g}}{1 \text{ mL}} = \dfrac{x \text{ g}}{100 \text{ mL}}$
b. x = 2 g of active ingredient in 100 mL of solution, therefore the percent strength is 2%.

Step 2: Calculate the percent concentration of lidocaine in the bag of NS.
a. 505 mL × x% = 5 mL × 2%
b. $505x = 10$
c. $x = 0.02$%

10. A
Step 1: 1000 mL × x% = 473 mL × 25%
Step 2: $1000x = 11{,}825$
Step 3: $x = 11.8$%

11. C
Step 1: 4% w/w × 1.06 × x mL = 2.5% w/v × 480 mL
Step 2: $4.24x = 1200$
Step 3: $x = 283$ mL

12. D
Step 1: Calculate the percent strength of the diluted solution.
a. 1892 mL × x% = 473 mL × 16%
b. $1892x = 7568$
c. $x = 4$%

Step 2: Calculate the ratio strength of the diluted solution.

a. $\dfrac{4}{100} = \dfrac{1\ \text{part}}{x\ \text{parts}}$

b. $4x = 100$

c. $x = 25$; therefore the ratio strength is 1:25.

13. B

Step 1: Calculate how many grams of potassium hydroxide are needed.

a. $\dfrac{1\ \text{g}}{5000\ \text{mL}} = \dfrac{x\ \text{g}}{120\ \text{mL}}$

b. $5000x = 120$

c. $x = 0.024\ \text{g}$

Step 2: Calculate how many milliliters of stock solution are needed to give 0.024 g of potassium hydroxide.

a. $\dfrac{4\ \text{g}}{100\ \text{mL}} = \dfrac{0.024\ \text{g}}{x\ \text{mL}}$

b. $4x = 2.4$

c. $x = 0.6\ \text{mL}$

14. C

Step 1: $2.5\% \times (x + 120\ \text{mL}) = 15\% \times 120\ \text{mL}$

Step 2: $2.5x + 300 = 1800$

Step 3: $2.5x = 1500$

Step 4: $x = 600\ \text{mL}$

15. B

Percentage		Parts
2.5%		1.75 parts
	1.75%	
0%		0.75 parts
		2.5 total parts

Quantity of 2.5% hydrocortisone ointment: 240 g × 1.75/2.5 = 168 g

Quantity of white petrolatum: 240 g × 0.75/2.5 = 72 g

16. C

Step 1: $85\%\ \text{w/w} \times 1.37 \times x\ \text{mL} = 25\%\ \text{w/v} \times 3785\ \text{mL}$

Step 2: $116.45x = 94{,}625$

Step 3: $x = 812.6\ \text{mL}$

17. D
Step 1: $40\% \times x\,g = 65\% \times 454\,g$
Step 2: $40x = 29{,}510$
Step 3: $x = 737.75\,g$

18. D
Step 1: $75\,g \times x\% = 60\,g \times 2\%$
Step 2: $75x = 120$
Step 3: $x = 1.6\%$

19. C
Step 1: $30\% \times x\,mL = 12\% \times 180\,mL$
Step 2: $30x = 2160$
Step 3: $x = 72\,mL$

20. D
Step 1: $2.5\% \times x\,mL = 0.75\% \times 240\,mL$
Step 2: $2.5x = 180\,mL$
Step 3: $x = 72\,mL$

21. D
Step 1: Calculate the amount of epinephrine in the diluted solution.
$750\,mL \times 1\,g/100\,mL = 7.5\,g$ of epinephrine in 750 milliliters of solution, which is also the amount in 30 milliliters of the stock solution.

Step 2: Calculate the amount of epinephrine needed to prepare 500 milliliters of a stock solution.
$500\,mL \times 7.5\,g/30\,mL = 125\,g$

22. B
$$\frac{\sum[(0.01\% \times 30\,g) + (0.025\% \times 70\,g) + (0.035\% \times 20\,g)]}{120\,g} = 0.023\%$$

23. B
Step 1: Convert the ratio strength of 1:80 w/v stock solution of sodium chloride to a percent strength.
a. $\dfrac{1\text{ part}}{80\text{ parts}} = \dfrac{x}{100}$
b. $80x = 100$
c. $x = 1.25$; therefore the percent strength is 1.25%

Step 2: Convert the ratio strength of 1:1000 w/v solution of sodium chloride to a percent strength.
a. $\dfrac{1\text{ part}}{1000\text{ parts}} = \dfrac{x}{100}$
b. $1000x = 100$
c. $x = 0.1$; therefore the percent strength is 0.1%

Step 3: Calculate how many milliliters of the 1:80 w/v stock solution of sodium chloride is required to prepare two liters of a 1:1000 w/v solution of sodium chloride.

a. $1.25\% \times x$ mL $= 0.1\% \times 2000$ mL

b. $1.25x = 200$

c. $x = 160$ mL

24. A

Percentage		Parts
40%		20 parts
	30%	
10%		10 parts
		30 total parts

Quantity of 10% urea cream: 180 g × 10/30 = 60 g

Quantity of 40% urea cream: 180 g × 20/30 = 120 g

25. B

Step 1: Calculate the percent strength of the 1:500 sodium chloride solution.

a. $\dfrac{1\text{ g}}{500\text{ mL}} = \dfrac{x\text{ g}}{100\text{ mL}}$

b. $500x = 100$

c. $x = 0.2$ g of active ingredient in 100 mL of solution, therefore the percent strength is 0.2%.

Step 2: Calculate how many milliliters of water must be added to the 1.75% sodium chloride solution to make a 1:500 sodium chloride solution.

a. $0.2\% \times (x + 60$ mL$) = 1.75\% \times 60$ mL

b. $0.2x + 12 = 105$

c. $0.2x = 93$

d. $x = 465$ mL

SECTION 8

PATIENT SPECIFIC DOSING

QUESTIONS

1. A child is to receive 25 mg/kg/day of cephalexin in divided doses every 8 hours. How many milligrams would a child weighing 44 pounds receive in each dose?

   a. 166.7 mg
   b. 240.1 mg
   c. 312.6 mg
   d. 366.7 mg

2. Calculate the body surface area for a patient that weighs 145 pounds and is 61 inches tall.

   a. 1.28 m²
   b. 1.47 m²
   c. 1.68 m²
   d. 1.93 m²

3. A physician orders lidocaine 1.5 mg/kg to be given to a patient weighing 200 pounds. The pharmacy has available lidocaine injection in a 4% solution. How many milliliters of the lidocaine solution will be needed for the patient?

   a. 1.7 mL
   b. 2.5 mL
   c. 2.8 mL
   d. 3.4 mL

4. A male patient that weighs 113 kilograms and is 5'9" tall is to receive tobramycin 2.5 mg/kg IV q12h. Calculate how many milligrams of tobramycin the patient would receive for each dose using his IBW.

   a. 153.24 mg
   b. 176.75 mg
   c. 192.55 mg
   d. 204.11 mg

5. A prescription calls for 20 mg/kg of a drug for a patient who weighs 198 pounds. How many milligrams of the drug should the patient receive?

   a. 1300 mg
   b. 1800 mg
   c. 2000 mg
   d. 2100 mg

6. A 67 year-old female who weighs 148 pounds is being started on cephalexin for the treatment of cellulitis. Her lab values are Na$^+$ 134 mEq/L, K$^+$ 4.7 mEq/L, BUN 26 mg/dL, and SCr 1.4 mg/dL. Using the chart below, what is the appropriate dose of cephalexin for this patient?

CrCl	≥ 60 mL/min	30-50 mL/min	15-29 mL/min	5-14 mL/min
Cephalexin Dose	500 mg q6h	500 mg q12h	250 mg q12h	250 mg q24h

a. 500 mg q6h
b. 500 mg q12h
c. 250 mg q12h
d. 250 mg q24h

7. A prescription calls for cisplatin 50 mg/m^2 per dose. How many milligrams of cisplatin are required for a patient that weighs 156 pounds and is 68 inches tall?

a. 92 mg
b. 115 mg
c. 128 mg
d. 147 mg

8. A child weighing 55 pounds is to receive 7 mg/kg of cefdinir twice daily. How many milligrams of cefdinir will the child receive per day?

a. 175 mg
b. 280 mg
c. 350 mg
d. 525 mg

9. A patient weighing 198 pounds is prescribed enoxaparin 1.5 mg/kg daily. The pharmacy has available prefilled syringes that have a concentration of 150 mg/mL. How many milliliters should be administered per day?

a. 0.6 mL
b. 0.9 mL
c. 1 mL
d. 1.5 mL

10. A prescription calls for 1.4 mg/m^2 of vincristine. The medication is available in an intravenous solution with a concentration of 0.75 mg/mL. How many milliliters are required for a patient that weighs 143 pounds and is 67 inches tall?

a. 2.19 mL
b. 2.45 mL
c. 3.27 mL
d. 3.86 mL

ANSWER KEY

1. A

$$44 \text{ lb} \times \frac{1 \text{ kg}}{2.2 \text{ lb}} \times \frac{25 \text{ kg}}{\text{mg/day}} \times \frac{1 \text{ day}}{3 \text{ doses}} = 166.7 \text{ mg/dose}$$

2. C

Step 1: 145 lb × 1 kg/2.2 lb = 65.91 kg

Step 2: 61 in × 2.54 cm/in = 154.94 cm

Step 3: $\sqrt{\dfrac{(154.94 \text{ cm} \times 65.91 \text{ kg})}{3600}} = 1.68 \text{ m}^2$

3. D

Step 1: Calculate how many grams of lidocaine are needed.

$$200 \text{ lb} \times \frac{1 \text{ kg}}{2.2 \text{ lb}} \times \frac{1.5 \text{ mg}}{1 \text{ kg}} \times \frac{1 \text{ g}}{1000 \text{ mg}} = 0.136 \text{ g}$$

Step 2: Calculate how many milliliters of lidocaine solution are needed.

a. $\dfrac{4 \text{ g}}{100 \text{ mL}} = \dfrac{0.136 \text{ g}}{x \text{ mL}}$

b. $4x = 13.6$

c. $x = 3.4$ mL

4. B

Step 1: Calculate the patient's IBW.
IBW (males) = 50 kg + (2.3 × 9) = 70.7 kg

Step 2: Calculate the dose of tobramycin the patient should receive.
2.5 mg/kg × 70.7 kg = 176.75 mg

5. B

$$198 \text{ lb} \times \frac{1 \text{ kg}}{2.2 \text{ lb}} \times \frac{20 \text{ mg}}{1 \text{ kg}} = 1800 \text{ mg}$$

6. B

Step 1: 148 lb × 1 kg/2.2 lb = 67.27 kg

Step 2: $\dfrac{(140 - 67) \times 67.27}{72 \times 1.4} \times 0.85 = 41.41$ mL/min, which corresponds to a cephalexin dose of 500 mg q12h.

7. A

Step 1: Calculate the patient's body surface area.

a. 156 lb × 1 kg/2.2 lb = 70.91 kg

b. 68 in × 2.54 cm/in = 172.72 cm

c. $\sqrt{\dfrac{(172.72 \text{ cm} \times 70.91 \text{ kg})}{3600}} = 1.84 \text{ m}^2$

Step 2: Calculate how many milligrams of cisplatin are required.
50 mg/m^2 × 1.84 m^2 = 92 mg

8. C

$$55 \text{ lb} \times \frac{1 \text{ kg}}{2.2 \text{ lb}} \times \frac{7 \text{ mg}}{\text{kg/dose}} \times \frac{2 \text{ doses}}{\text{day}} = 350 \text{ mg/day}$$

9. B

Step 1: Calculate how many milligrams of enoxaparin are needed.

$$198 \text{ lb} \times \frac{1 \text{ kg}}{2.2 \text{ lb}} \times \frac{1.5 \text{ kg}}{1 \text{ kg}} = 135 \text{ mg}$$

Step 2: Calculate how many milliliters of enoxaparin are needed.
135 mg × 1 mL/150 mg = 0.9 mL

10. C

Step 1: Calculate the patient's body surface area.

a. 143 lb × 1 kg/2.2 lb = 65 kg

b. 67 in × 2.54 cm/in = 170.18 cm

c. $\sqrt{\dfrac{(170.18 \text{ cm} \times 65 \text{ kg})}{3600}} = 1.75 \text{ m}^2$

Step 2: Calculate how many milligrams of vincristine are required.
1.4 mg/m^2 × 1.75 m^2 = 2.45 mg

Step 3: Calculate how many milliliters of vincristine intravenous solution are required.
2.45 mg × 1 mL/0.75 mg = 3.27 mL

SECTION 9

COMPOUNDING

QUESTIONS

1. Calculate how many grams of losartan are required for the following prescription.

Rx:
Losartan
Hydrochlorothiazide aa 50 mg
Dispense 14 charts
Sig: i chart qd ud

a. 0.7 g
b. 1.3 g
c. 1.8 g
d. 2.6 g

2. A pharmacist is to prepare an oral solution formulation of the following compound and has available a codeine injection with a concentration of 60 mg/2 mL. Calculate how many milliliters of the codeine injection solution are needed to prepare the following prescription.

Rx:
Codeine 20 mg/5 mL
Dispense 180 mL
Sig: 5 mL q4h prn

a. 9 mL
b. 17 mL
c. 20 mL
d. 24 mL

3. A medication order calls for 2.5 mg/kg of tobramycin to be added to 250 milliliters of D5W for a patient that weighs 165 pounds. How many milliliters of a tobramycin injection with a concentration of 80 mg/2 mL should be used to prepare the infusion?

a. 2.41 mL
b. 3.89 mL
c. 4.17 mL
d. 4.69 mL

4. Calculate how many grams of 2.5% ointment can be made from 32 grams of salicylic acid.

a. 1153 g
b. 1280 g
c. 1297 g
d. 1340 g

The following information relates to questions 5 – 6.

An intravenous infusion is to contain 20 milliequivalents of potassium ion and 25 milliequivalents of sodium ion in 250 milliliters of D5W. The pharmacy has available potassium chloride injection that has a concentration of 5 g/30 mL and 0.9% sodium chloride injection.

5. How many milliliters of potassium chloride injection should be used to make the infusion? (M.W. of KCl = 74.5)

   a. 6.87 mL
   b. 8.25 mL
   c. 8.94 mL
   d. 12.76 mL

6. How many milliliters of sodium chloride injection should be used to make the infusion? (M.W. of NaCl = 58.4)

   a. 149.3 mL
   b. 162.2 mL
   c. 178.1 mL
   d. 180.6 mL

7. A dropper is calibrated to deliver 20 drops of LCD per milliliter. How many drops are required for a prescription compound calling for 2.75 milliliters of LCD?

   a. 25 gtts
   b. 37 gtts
   c. 40 gtts
   d. 55 gtts

8. How many milliliters of an injection containing 100 milligrams of lidocaine per milliliter should be used to prepare the following prescription?

   Rx:
   Lidocaine   3%
   Aquaphor   qs 60 g
   Sig: apply as directed

   a. 8 mL
   b. 10 mL
   c. 13 mL
   d. 18 mL

The following prescription relates to questions 9 – 12.

Rx:
Menthol crystals
Camphor crystals   aa 0.5%
Salicylic acid powder   2%
Cerave   qs 120 g

9. Calculate how many grams of menthol crystals are needed.

    a. 0.6 g
    b. 0.75 g
    c. 1.2 g
    d. 1.45 g

10. Calculate how many grams of camphor crystals are needed.

    a. 0.3 g
    b. 0.6 g
    c. 1.2 g
    d. 1.4 g

11. Calculate how many grams of salicylic acid powder are needed.

    a. 0.8 g
    b. 1.5 g
    c. 1.9 g
    d. 2.4 g

12. Calculate how many grams of Cerave are needed.

    a. 100.9 g
    b. 105.8 g
    c. 110.3 g
    d. 116.4 g

13. A prescription calls for 0.7 grams of sodium chloride to be dissolved in purified water to form a solution. If the solubility of sodium chloride in water is 1 g/2.8 mL, how many milliliters of water are required to dissolve the sodium chloride?

    a. 0.9 mL
    b. 1.52 mL
    c. 1.96 mL
    d. 2.14 mL

14. How many milligrams of naphazoline hydrochloride are needed to compound the following prescription?

Rx:
Naphazoline HCl 0.05%
Dispense 15 mL
Sig: 1 spray in each nostril bid

a. 3.8 mg
b. 4.2 mg
c. 7.5 mg
d. 10.5 mg

15. Calculate the how many grams of Polybase are required to compound 100 suppositories from the following formula for one progesterone vaginal suppository.

Progesterone, micronized	20 mg
Lactose	15 mg
Polybase	qs 2 g

a. 189 g
b. 196.5 g
c. 200 g
d. 210.5 g

16. Calculate how many captopril tablets (100 mg each) will be needed to compound the following prescription.

Rx:
Captopril 25 mg/5 mL
Dispense 2 week supply
Sig: i tsp po bid

a. 5 tablets
b. 7 tablets
c. 10 tablets
d. 14 tablets

17. How many milliliters of an injection containing 1 gram of drug in 5 milliliters should be used to fill a medication order that requires 350 milligrams of the drug to be added to 500 milliliters of NS?

a. 1.75 mL
b. 2.54 mL
c. 3.65 mL
d. 4.18 mL

The following prescription relates to questions 18 – 21.

Rx:
Prednisone 0.75 mg
Dispense 15 charts
Sig: 1 chart bid

18. Calculate how many milligrams of prednisone are required for the prescription.

    a. 11.25 mg
    b. 11.75 mg
    c. 12.25 mg
    d. 12.5 mg

19. If prednisone 5 milligram tablets are available, how many tablets must be used to compound the prescription? (Round answer to the nearest whole number.)

    a. 3 tablets
    b. 5 tablets
    c. 6 tablets
    d. 8 tablets

20. The amount of tablets calculated in question 19 are crushed and weigh 300 milligrams. How many milligrams of the crushed tablets are required for the prescription?

    a. 115 mg
    b. 145 mg
    c. 180 mg
    d. 225 mg

21. The total desired weight for each chart is 180 milligrams. How many milligrams of lactose should be used as a diluent to prepare the entire prescription?

    a. 2400 mg
    b. 2475 mg
    c. 2560 mg
    d. 2585 mg

22. Calculate how many milligrams of testosterone are needed to compound the following prescription. The source of testosterone to be used is a 100 mg/g trituration.

Rx:
Testosterone   2 mg/mL
Ethoxy diglycol   3 mL
Hydrogel   qs 30 mL
Sig: apply bid ud

a. 0.5 g
b. 0.6 g
c. 1.1 g
d. 1.4 g

23. Calculate how many grams of hydrochlorothiazide are required for the following prescription.

Rx:
Losartan
Hydrochlorothiazide   aa qs 25 mg
Dispense 30 charts
Sig: i chart qd ud

a. 0.25 g
b. 0.375 g
c. 0.515 g
d. 0.75 g

24. How many grams of guaifenesin are required to compound the following prescription?

Rx:
Dextromethorphan syrup 15 mg/mL   30 mL
Guaifenesin   200 mg/10 mL
Cherry Syrup   qs 120 mL
Sig: 1 tsp q6h prn

a. 0.9 g
b. 1.7 g
c. 2 g
d. 2.4 g

25. Calculate how many grams of codeine powder are required to compound the following prescription.

Rx:
Codeine 20 mg capsules
Dispense 60 caps
Sig: i cap q4h prn

a. 0.8 g
b. 1.2 g
c. 1.5 g
d. 2.2 g

ANSWER KEY

1. A
14 charts × 50 mg/chart = 700 mg ÷ 1000 = 0.7 g

2. D
Step 1: Calculate how many milligrams of codeine are needed.
20 mg/5 mL × 180 mL = 720 mg

Step 2: Calculate how many milliliters of codeine injection are needed.
a. $\dfrac{60 \text{ mg}}{2 \text{ mL}} = \dfrac{720 \text{ mg}}{x \text{ mL}}$
b. $60x = 1440$
c. $x = 24$ mL

3. D
Step 1: Calculate how many milligrams of tobramycin are needed.
$165 \text{ lb} \times \dfrac{1 \text{ kg}}{2.2 \text{ lb}} \times \dfrac{2.5 \text{ mg}}{1 \text{ kg}} = 187.5 \text{ mg}$

Step 2: Calculate how many milliliters of tobramycin injection are needed.
a. $\dfrac{80 \text{ mg}}{2 \text{ mL}} = \dfrac{187.5 \text{ mg}}{x \text{ mL}}$
b. $80x = 375$
c. $x = 4.69$ mL

4. B
Step 1: $\dfrac{2.5 \text{ g}}{100 \text{ g}} = \dfrac{32 \text{ g}}{x \text{ g}}$
Step 2: $2.5x = 3200$
Step 3: $x = 1280$ g

5. C
$20 \text{ mEq} \times \dfrac{74.5 \text{ mg}}{1 \text{ mEq}} \times \dfrac{1 \text{ g}}{1000 \text{ mg}} \times \dfrac{30 \text{ mL}}{5 \text{ g}} = 8.94 \text{ mL}$

6. B
$25 \text{ mEq} \times \dfrac{58.4 \text{ mg}}{1 \text{ mEq}} \times \dfrac{1 \text{ g}}{1000 \text{ mg}} \times \dfrac{100 \text{ mL}}{0.9 \text{ g}} = 162.2 \text{ mL}$

7. D
2.75 mL × 20 gtts/mL = 55 gtts

8. D
Step 1: Calculate how many milligrams of lidocaine are needed.
0.03 × 60 g = 1.8 g × 1000 = 1800 mg

Step 2: Calculate how many milliliters of lidocaine injection are needed.

a. $\dfrac{100\text{ mg}}{1\text{ mL}} = \dfrac{1800\text{ mg}}{x\text{ mL}}$

b. $100x = 1800$

c. $x = 18$ mL

9. A
0.005 × 120 g = 0.6 g

10. B
0.005 × 120 g = 0.6 g

11. D
0.02 × 120 g = 2.4 g

12. D
120 g – (0.6 g + 0.6 g + 2.4 g) = 116.4 g

13. C
0.7 g × 2.8 mL/g = 1.96 mL

14. C
Step 1: $\dfrac{0.05\text{ g}}{100\text{ mL}} = \dfrac{x\text{ g}}{15\text{ mL}}$

Step 2: $100x = 0.75$

Step 3: $x = 0.0075$ g × 1000 = 7.5 mg

15. B
Step 1: Calculate how many grams of Polybase are required for one suppository.
2 g – (0.02 g + 0.015 g) = 1.965 g

Step 2: Calculate how many grams of Polybase are required for 100 suppositories.
1.965 g/suppository × 100 suppositories = 196.5 g

16. B
Step 1: Calculate how many milliliters are required for the prescription.

$\dfrac{5\text{ mL}}{\text{dose}} \times \dfrac{2\text{ doses}}{\text{day}} \times 14\text{ days} = 140$ mL

Step 2: Calculate how many milligrams of captopril are required for the prescription.
140 mL × 25 mg/5 mL = 700 mg

Step 3: Calculate the number of captopril 50 mg tablets that are required for the prescription.

a. $\dfrac{1\ \text{tab}}{100\ \text{mg}} = \dfrac{x\ \text{tabs}}{700\ \text{mg}}$

b. $100x = 700$

c. $x = 7$ tablets

17. A

Step 1: $\dfrac{1000\ \text{mg}}{5\ \text{mL}} = \dfrac{350\ \text{mg}}{x\ \text{mL}}$

Step 2: $1000x = 1750$

Step 3: $x = 1.75$ mL

18. A

15 charts × 0.75 mg/chart = 11.25 mg

19. A

Step 1: Calculate how many milligrams of prednisone are required.

15 charts × 0.75 mg/chart = 11.25 mg

Step 2: Calculate the number of prednisone 5 mg tablets that are required.

a. $\dfrac{1\ \text{tab}}{5\ \text{mg}} = \dfrac{x\ \text{tabs}}{11.25\ \text{mg}}$

b. $5x = 11.25$

c. $x = 2.25$ tablets = 3 tablets

20. D

a. $\dfrac{3\ \text{tabs}}{300\ \text{mg}} = \dfrac{2.25\ \text{tabs}}{x\ \text{mg}}$

b. $3x = 675$

c. $x = 225$ mg of crushed tablets

21. B

Step 1: Calculate the total weight of 15 charts.

180 mg/chart × 15 charts = 2700 mg

Step 2: Calculate the amount of lactose that should be used.

2700 mg (total weight) – 225 mg (crushed tablet weight) = 2475 mg

22. B

Step 1: Calculate the amount of testosterone needed.

2 mg/mL × 30 mL = 60 mg

Step 2: Calculate how many milligrams of the trituration are needed.

a. $\dfrac{100\ mg}{1\ g} = \dfrac{60\ mg}{x\ g}$

b. $100x = 60$

c. $x = 0.6\ g$

23. B

30 charts × 12.5 mg/chart = 375 mg ÷ 1000 = 0.375 g

24. D

Step 1: $\dfrac{200\ mg}{10\ mL} = \dfrac{x\ mg}{120\ mL}$

Step 2: $10x = 24{,}000$

Step 3: $x = 2400\ mg ÷ 1000 = 2.4\ g$

25. B

20 mg/cap × 60 caps = 1200 mg ÷ 1000 = 1.2 g

SECTION 10

EXPRESSIONS OF CONCENTRATION

QUESTIONS

1. How many milligrams of hydrocortisone are in 60 grams of a 1.5% cream?

   a. 275 mg
   b. 525 mg
   c. 650 mg
   d. 900 mg

2. A pharmacist adds 180 milliliters of acetic acid to water to prepare a total volume of 3 quarts. Calculate the percent strength (v/v) of acetic acid.

   a. 4.7%
   b. 5.9%
   c. 6.3%
   d. 10.8%

3. A patient's blood glucose level was determined to be 284 mg%. How many grams of glucose are in one liter of the patient's blood?

   a. 0.81 g
   b. 2.84 g
   c. 4.97 g
   d. 5.32 g

4. Calculate the percent strength (v/v) of alcohol for the following prescription.

Rx:
30% v/v alcohol	600 mL
60% v/v alcohol	900 mL
Glycerin	qs ad 2500 mL

   a. 21.3%
   b. 25.4%
   c. 28.8%
   d. 36.5%

5. Express 0.0042% w/v as parts per million.

   a. 0.42 ppm
   b. 4.2 ppm
   c. 42 ppm
   d. 420 ppm

6. How many milligrams of dextrose are in 750 milliliters of D50W?

    a. 375 mg
    b. 3750 mg
    c. 37,500 mg
    d. 375,000 mg

7. Convert 1:4500 to a percent strength.

    a. 0.002%
    b. 0.02%
    c. 0.2%
    d. 2%

8. One pint of an active ingredient is diluted to two liters. Calculate the percent strength (v/v).

    a. 16.57%
    b. 23.65%
    c. 28.94%
    d. 35.44%

9. Calculate how many milligrams of potassium permanganate are needed for the following prescription.

Rx:
Potassium permanganate 1:6500
Dispense 1 quart
Sig: use daily as directed

    a. 98 mg
    b. 103 mg
    c. 127 mg
    d. 146 mg

10. Convert 0.25% to a ratio strength.

    a. 1:40
    b. 1:400
    c. 1:4000
    d. 1:40,000

11. **A pharmacist dissolves 1250 milligrams of dextrose in 30 milliliters of water. What is the percent strength (w/w) of the solution?**

    a. 4%
    b. 6.5%
    c. 7%
    d. 8.5%

12. **Calculate the percent strength (w/w) of hydrocortisone for the following prescription.**

    Rx:
    Hydrocortisone 2.5% cream   5 g
    Lidocaine   10 g
    Cerave   30 g

    a. 0.13%
    b. 0.28 %
    c. 0.47%
    d. 0.81%

13. **The tested level of lead in drinking water was measured to be 6.8 ppm. How many milligrams of lead are present in 20 gallons of water?**

    a. 515 mg
    b. 575 mg
    c. 680 mg
    d. 720 mg

14. **One quart of lotion contains 75 milliliters of benzyl alcohol. Calculate the percent strength (v/v) of benzyl alcohol in the lotion.**

    a. 3.62%
    b. 5.84%
    c. 6.95%
    d. 7.93%

15. **A pharmacist dissolves 250 milligrams of sucrose in enough water to make 1 liter of solution. Calculate the percent strength (w/v) of sucrose in the solution.**

    a. 0.025%
    b. 0.75%
    c. 1.25%
    d. 1.5%

16. Convert 1:2000 to a percent strength.

    a. 0.05%
    b. 0.5%
    c. 5%
    d. 50%

17. Calculate how many grams of benzalkonium chloride must be dissolved in 300 milliliters of glycerin (SG = 1.25) to make a 15% w/w solution.

    a. 42.35 g
    b. 56.25 g
    c. 66.18 g
    d. 74.29 g

18. How many milligrams of sodium chloride are in 1.5 liters of normal saline?

    a. 135 mg
    b. 1350 mg
    c. 13,500 mg
    d. 135,000 mg

19. Calculate how many milliliters of a 6% w/v stock solution of potassium hydroxide should be used to compound the following prescription.

Rx:
Potassium hydroxide solution 1:2500
Dispense 180 mL
Sig: use as directed

    a. 0.9 mL
    b. 1.2 mL
    c. 1.6 mL
    d. 2.3 mL

20. 120 grams of an ointment contains 8 grams of an active ingredient. Calculate the percent strength (w/w) of the active ingredient in the ointment.

    a. 6.67%
    b. 8.93%
    c. 10.86%
    d. 15.47%

21. If 120 grams of tannic acid are dissolved in 1500 milliliters of water, what is the percent strength (w/w) of the solution?

   a. 7.4%
   b. 9.2%
   c. 13.6%
   d. 17.9%

22. Convert 6.25% to a ratio strength.

   a. 1:16
   b. 1:160
   c. 1:1600
   d. 1:16,000

23. Calculate the percent strength (w/w) of ketoconazole in a preparation made by adding 10 grams of ketoconazole to 100 grams of 2% ketoconazole cream.

   a. 5.7%
   b. 8.2%
   c. 9.1%
   d. 10.9%

24. A pharmacist dissolves 4.5 grams of menthol in 120 milliliters of alcohol. What is the percent strength (w/v) of the solution? (The specific gravity of alcohol is 0.812 and the specific gravity of the solution is 0.98.)

   a. 3.75%
   b. 4.32%
   c. 4.41%
   d. 7.63%

25. One quart of a solution contains 2500 milligrams of an active ingredient. Calculate the percent strength (w/v).

   a. 0.12%
   b. 0.17%
   c. 0.26%
   d. 0.48%

ANSWER KEY

1. D

Step 1: $\dfrac{1.5\text{ g}}{100\text{ g}} = \dfrac{x\text{ g}}{60\text{ g}}$

Step 2: $100x = 90$

Step 3: $x = 0.90\text{ g} \times 1000 = 900\text{ mg}$

2. C

Step 1: $\dfrac{180\text{ mL}}{2838\text{ mL}} = \dfrac{x\text{ mL}}{100\text{ mL}}$

Step 2: $2838x = 18,000$

Step 3: $x = 6.3$ mL of acetic acid in 100 mL of solution, therefore the percent strength is 6.3%.

3. B

Step 1: $\dfrac{284\text{ mg}}{100\text{ mL}} = \dfrac{x\text{ mg}}{1000\text{ mL}}$

Step 2: $100x = 284,000$

Step 3: $x = 2840\text{ mg} \div 1000 = 2.84\text{ g}$

4. C

$$\dfrac{\sum[(30\% \times 600\text{ mL}) + (60\% \times 900\text{ mL}) + (0\% \times 1000\text{ mL})]}{2500\text{ mL}} = 28.8\%$$

5. C

Step 1: $\dfrac{0.0042\text{ g}}{100\text{ mL}} = \dfrac{x\text{ g}}{1,000,000}$

Step 2: $100x = 4200$

Step 3: $x = 42$ ppm

6. D

Step 1: $\dfrac{50\text{ g}}{100\text{ mL}} = \dfrac{x\text{ g}}{750\text{ mL}}$

Step 2: $100x = 37,500$

Step 3: $x = 375\text{ g} \times 1000 = 375,000\text{ mg}$

7. B

Step 1: $\dfrac{1\text{ part}}{4500\text{ parts}} = \dfrac{x}{100}$

Step 2: $4500x = 100$

Step 3: $x = 0.02$; therefore the percent strength is 0.02%.

8. B

Step 1: $\dfrac{473 \text{ mL}}{2000 \text{ mL}} = \dfrac{x \text{ mL}}{100 \text{ mL}}$

Step 2: $2000x = 47{,}300$

Step 3: $x = 23.65$ mL of active ingredient in 100 mL of solution, therefore the percent strength is 23.65%.

9. D

Step 1: $\dfrac{1 \text{ g}}{6500 \text{ mL}} = \dfrac{x \text{ g}}{946 \text{ mL}}$

Step 2: $6500x = 946$ mL

Step 3: $x = 0.146$ g $\times$ 1000 = 146 mg

10. B

Step 1: $\dfrac{0.25}{100} = \dfrac{1 \text{ part}}{x \text{ parts}}$

Step 2: $0.25x = 100$

Step 3: $x = 400$; therefore the ratio strength is 1:400.

11. A

$\dfrac{1.25 \text{ g}}{1.25 \text{ g} + 30 \text{ g}} \times 100 = 4\%$

12. B

Step 1: Calculate the amount of hydrocortisone in the prescription.

a. $\dfrac{2.5 \text{ g}}{100 \text{ g}} = \dfrac{x \text{ g}}{5 \text{ g}}$

b. $100x = 12.5$

c. $x = 0.125$ g

Step 2: Calculate the total weight of the prescription.
5 g + 10 g + 30 g = 45 g

Step 3: Calculate the percent strength of hydrocortisone in the final preparation.

a. $\dfrac{0.125 \text{ g}}{45 \text{ g}} = \dfrac{x \text{ g}}{100 \text{ g}}$

b. $45x = 12.5$

c. $x = 0.28$ g of hydrocortisone in 100 g of cream, therefore the percent strength is 0.28%.

13. A

Step 1: $\dfrac{6.8 \text{ g}}{1{,}000{,}000} = \dfrac{x \text{ g}}{75{,}700 \text{ mL}}$

Step 2: $1{,}000{,}000x = 514{,}760$

Step 3: $x = 0.515$ g $\times$ 1000 = 515 mg

14. D

Step 1: $\dfrac{75 \text{ mL}}{946 \text{ mL}} = \dfrac{x \text{ mL}}{100 \text{ mL}}$

Step 2: $946x = 7500$

Step 3: $x = 7.93$ mL of benzyl alcohol in 100 mL of lotion, therefore the percent strength is 7.93%.

15. A

Step 1: $\dfrac{0.25 \text{ g}}{1000 \text{ mL}} = \dfrac{x \text{ g}}{100 \text{ mL}}$

Step 2: $1000x = 25$

Step 3: $x = 0.025$ g of sucrose in 100 mL of solution, therefore the percent strength is 0.025%.

16. A

Step 1: $\dfrac{1 \text{ part}}{2000 \text{ parts}} = \dfrac{x}{100}$

Step 2: $2000x = 100$

Step 3: $x = 0.05$; therefore the percent strength is 0.05%.

17. C

Step 1: Calculate the weight of the glycerin.
300 mL × 1.25 = 375 g

Step 2: Calculate how many grams of benzalkonium chloride are needed.

a. $\dfrac{x \text{ g}}{x \text{ g} + 375 \text{ g}} = \dfrac{15 \text{ g}}{100 \text{ g}}$

b. $100x = 15x + 5625$

c. $85x = 5625$

d. $x = 66.18$ g

18. C

Step 1: $\dfrac{0.9 \text{ g}}{100 \text{ mL}} = \dfrac{x \text{ g}}{1500 \text{ mL}}$

Step 2: $100x = 1350$

Step 3: $x = 13.5$ g × 1000 = 13,500 mg

19. B

Step 1: Calculate how many grams of potassium hydroxide are needed.

a. $\dfrac{1 \text{ g}}{2500 \text{ mL}} = \dfrac{x \text{ g}}{180 \text{ mL}}$

b. $2500x = 180$

c. $x = 0.072$ g

Step 2: Calculate how many milliliters of stock solution are needed to give 0.072 g of potassium hydroxide.

a. $\dfrac{6\ \text{g}}{100\ \text{mL}} = \dfrac{0.072\ \text{g}}{x\ \text{mL}}$

b. $6x = 7.2$

c. $x = 1.2\ \text{mL}$

20. A

Step 1: $\dfrac{8\ \text{g}}{120\ \text{g}} = \dfrac{x\ \text{g}}{100\ \text{g}}$

Step 2: $120x = 800$

Step 3: $x = 6.67$ g of active ingredient in 100 g of ointment, therefore the percent strength is 6.67%.

21. A

$\dfrac{120\ \text{g}}{120\ \text{g} + 1500\ \text{g}} \times 100 = 7.4\%$

22. A

Step 1: $\dfrac{6.25}{100} = \dfrac{1\ \text{part}}{x\ \text{parts}}$

Step 2: $6.25x = 100$

Step 3: $x = 16$; therefore the ratio strength is 1:16.

23. D

$\dfrac{10\ \text{g} + 2\ \text{g}}{10\ \text{g} + 100\ \text{g}} \times 100 = 10.9\%$

24. B

Step 1: Calculate the weight of the alcohol.
$120\ \text{mL} \times 0.812 = 97.44$ g

Step 2: Calculate the w/w% of the solution.

$\dfrac{4.5\ \text{g}}{4.5\ \text{g} + 97.44\ \text{g}} \times 100 = 4.41\%\ \text{w/w}$

Step 3: Calculate the w/v% of the solution.
$4.41\%\ \text{w/w} \times 0.98 = 4.32\%\ \text{w/v}$

25. C

Step 1: $\dfrac{2.5\ \text{g}}{946\ \text{mL}} = \dfrac{x\ \text{g}}{100\ \text{mL}}$

Step 2: $946x = 250$

Step 3: $x = 0.26$ g of active ingredient in 100 mL of solution, therefore the percent strength is 0.26%.

SECTION 11

NUTRITION SUPPORT

QUESTIONS

1. A patient weighing 90 kilograms is to receive the following TPN prescription. Calculate how many grams of protein the patient will receive per day.

Rx:
Amino acids   4.5% (final concentration)
Dextrose   25% (final concentration)
Rate: 130 mL/hr

    a. 108.5 g
    b. 115.6 g
    c. 121.2 g
    d. 140.4 g

2. A patient weighing 78 kilograms has a caloric requirement of 2150 calories per day. The TPN formula she is to receive has a caloric density of 0.92 cal/mL. Calculate the infusion rate in mL/hr if the TPN is to be infused over 24 hours. (Round answer to the nearest whole number.)

    a. 97 mL/hr
    b. 106 mL/hr
    c. 115 mL/hr
    d. 122 mL/hr

The following TPN order relates to questions 3 – 12.

Item	Quantity	Available Supplies
Amino Acids 8.5%	500 mL	Amino Acids 8.5%
Dextrose 50%	450 mL	Dextrose 50%
Sodium Chloride	35 mEq	NaCl 4 mEq/mL
Potassium Chloride	20 mEq	KCl 2 mEq/mL
Calcium Gluconate	5 mEq	Calcium Gluconate 0.465 mEq/mL
Magnesium Sulfate	8 mEq	Magnesium Sulfate 4.06 mEq/mL
MVI-12	5 mL	MVI-12 10 mL vial
Trace Elements	2 mL	Trace Elements 5 mL vial

3. Calculate how many milliliters of sodium chloride are required.

    a. 8.75 mL
    b. 9.1 mL
    c. 11.25 mL
    d. 12.5 mL

4. Calculate how many milliliters of potassium chloride are required.

    a. 2 mL
    b. 5 mL
    c. 7 mL
    d. 10 mL

5. Calculate how many milliliters of calcium gluconate are required.

    a. 8.5 mL
    b. 10.75 mL
    c. 12.45 mL
    d. 13.25 mL

6. Calculate how many milliliters of magnesium sulfate are required.

    a. 1.97 mL
    b. 2.54 mL
    c. 4.83 mL
    d. 5.21 mL

7. Calculate the total volume of the final TPN solution. (Round answer to the nearest whole number.)

    a. 970 mL
    b. 988 mL
    c. 1026 mL
    d. 1077 mL

8. Calculate the flow rate in mL/hr if the entire TPN bag is to be infused over 18 hours. (Round answer to the nearest whole number.)

    a. 55 mL/hr
    b. 58 mL/hr
    c. 63 mL/hr
    d. 70 mL/hr

9. How many total calories will the patient receive from the TPN solution?

    a. 827 kcal
    b. 856 kcal
    c. 935 kcal
    d. 1118 kcal

10. **Calculate the percentage of the total calories of the TPN that are represented by the protein component. (Round answer to the nearest whole number.)**

    a. 18%
    b. 20%
    c. 21%
    d. 29%

11. **Calculate the percentage of the total calories of the TPN that are represented by the dextrose component. (Round answer to the nearest whole number.)**

    a. 71%
    b. 82%
    c. 85%
    d. 87%

12. **Calculate the grams of nitrogen contained in the TPN.**

    a. 4.9 g
    b. 5.3 g
    c. 6.4 g
    d. 6.8 g

13. **Calculate the BMI for a patient that weighs 190 pounds and is 6'4" tall.**

    a. 22.6
    b. 23.2
    c. 25.6
    d. 26.1

14. **A patient is receiving 320 milliliters of 10% lipid emulsion. How many calories is the patient receiving from the lipid emulsion?**

    a. 275 kcal
    b. 320 kcal
    c. 352 kcal
    d. 467 kcal

15. **A patient is receiving 85 grams of protein from a 10% amino acid injection solution. How many calories are provided by the solution?**

    a. 85 kcal
    b. 170 kcal
    c. 298 kcal
    d. 340 kcal

16. A patient weighing 68 kilograms is to receive the following TPN prescription. Calculate how much fluid the patient will receive per day in liters.

Rx:
Amino acids   3.5% (final concentration)
Dextrose   20% (final concentration)
Rate: 160 mL/hr

a. 3.52 L
b. 3.84 L
c. 3.99 L
d. 4.13 L

17. Calculate the non-protein caloric requirement for a 59 year old female with a calculated BEE (basal energy expenditure) of 1200 calories, a stress factor of 1.4, and an activity factor of 1.3.

a. 1560 kcal
b. 1680 kcal
c. 1833 kcal
d. 2184 kcal

18. A patient has a TEE (total energy expenditure) of 2275 kcal/day. The patient is receiving 780 calories from protein and 1400 calories from dextrose. How many calories should be provided by the lipids?

a. 875 kcal
b. 1064 kcal
c. 1237 kcal
d. 1495 kcal

19. A 72 year old male who weighs 155 pounds and is 5'9" tall is to receive 1.5 g/kg/day of protein. Calculate his daily protein requirement using his actual weight.

a. 46.9 g
b. 82.5 g
c. 105.7 g
d. 110.3 g

20. A patient is receiving 580 milliliters of D50W in her TPN per day. How many calories are provided by the D50W?

a. 872 kcal
b. 986 kcal
c. 1160 kcal
d. 1239 kcal

21. A patient is to receive 415 calories provided by lipids. The concentration of the lipid emulsion available is 20%. How many milliliters of the lipid emulsion are required?

   a. 207.5 mL
   b. 310.8 mL
   c. 377.3 mL
   d. 405.1 mL

22. A pharmacy receives the following TPN order. Calculate how many milliliters of dextrose 20% should be added to the TPN. (Round answer to the nearest whole number.)

Item	Quantity	Available Supplies
Amino Acids 7.5%	55 g	Amino Acids 7.5%
Dextrose 20%	395 g	Dextrose 20%
Sodium Chloride	35 mEq	NaCl 4 mEq/mL
Potassium Chloride	20 mEq	KCl 2 mEq/mL
Calcium Gluconate	4.65 mEq	Calcium Gluconate 0.465 mEq/mL
Magnesium Sulfate	8 mEq	Magnesium Sulfate 4.06 mEq/mL
MVI-12	5 mL	MVI-12 10 mL vial
Trace Elements	2 mL	Trace Elements 5 mL vial

   a. 1552 mL
   b. 1691 mL
   c. 1742 mL
   d. 1975 mL

23. Using the Harris-Benedict equation, calculate the BEE (basal energy expenditure) for a 71 year old male patient who weighs 210 pounds and is 6'1" tall. (Round answer to the nearest whole number.)

   a. 1826 kcal
   b. 1914 kcal
   c. 1993 kcal
   d. 2137 kcal

24. A pharmacist is preparing a TPN order for 180 grams of dextrose. The concentration of dextrose available is 30%. How many milliliters of dextrose are required?

   a. 480 mL
   b. 600 mL
   c. 675 mL
   d. 810 mL

25. A patient weighing 82 kilograms is to receive the following TPN prescription. Calculate how many grams of dextrose the patient will receive per day.

Rx:
Amino acids   4% (final concentration)
Dextrose   25% (final concentration)
Rate: 140 mL/hr

a. 700 g
b. 737 g
c. 840 g
d. 896 g

ANSWER KEY

1. D
Step 1: Calculate the number of milliliters of TPN the patient will receive per day.
130 mL/hr × 24 hr = 3120 mL

Step 2: Calculate how many grams of protein the patient will receive per day.

a. $\dfrac{4.5\ g}{100\ mL} = \dfrac{x\ g}{3120\ mL}$

b. $100x = 14{,}040$

c. $x = 140.4\ g$

2. A
$\dfrac{2150\ cal}{day} \times \dfrac{1\ mL}{0.92\ cal} \times \dfrac{1\ day}{24\ hr} = 97.4\ mL/hr = 97\ mL/hr$

3. A
1 mL/4 mEq × 35 mEq = 8.75 mL

4. D
1 mL/2 mEq × 20 mEq = 10 mL

5. B
1 mL/0.465 mEq × 5 mEq = 10.75 mL

6. A
1 mL/4.06 mEq × 8 mEq = 1.97 mL

7. B
Step 1: Calculate the quantity required for each ingredient.
a. Quantity of amino acids: 500 mL
b. Quantity of dextrose: 450 mL
c. Quantity of sodium chloride: 1 mL/4 mEq × 35 mEq = 8.75 mL
d. Quantity of potassium chloride: 1 mL/2 mEq × 20 mEq = 10 mL
e. Quantity of calcium gluconate: 1 mL/0.465 mEq × 5 mEq = 10.75 mL
f. Quantity of magnesium sulfate: 1 mL/4.06 mEq × 8 mEq = 1.97 mL
g. Quantity of MVI-12: 5 mL
h. Quantity of trace elements: 2 mL

Step 2: Calculate the sum of all ingredients from step 1.
500 mL + 450 mL + 8.75 mL + 10 mL + 10.75 mL + 1.97 mL + 5 mL + 2 mL = 988.47 mL
= 988 mL

8. A
988 mL/18 hr = 54.9 mL/hr = 55 mL/hr

9. C

Step 1: Calculate the calories from the amino acids.

a. $\dfrac{8.5 \text{ g}}{100 \text{ mL}} = \dfrac{x \text{ g}}{500 \text{ mL}}$

b. $100x = 4250$

c. $x = 42.5 \text{ g}$

d. $42.5 \text{ g} \times 4 \text{ kcal/g} = 170 \text{ kcal}$

Step 2: Calculate the calories from the dextrose.

a. $\dfrac{50 \text{ g}}{100 \text{ mL}} = \dfrac{x \text{ g}}{450 \text{ mL}}$

b. $100x = 22{,}500$

c. $x = 225 \text{ g}$

d. $225 \text{ g} \times 3.4 \text{ kcal/g} = 765 \text{ kcal}$

Step 3: Calculate the sum of calories from the amino acids (step 1) and dextrose (step 2).
170 kcal + 765 kcal = 935 kcal

10. A

Step 1: Calculate the calories from the amino acids.

a. $\dfrac{8.5 \text{ g}}{100 \text{ mL}} = \dfrac{x \text{ g}}{500 \text{ mL}}$

b. $100x = 4250$

c. $x = 42.5 \text{ g}$

d. $42.5 \text{ g} \times 4 \text{ kcal/g} = 170 \text{ kcal}$

Step 2: Calculate the calories from the dextrose.

a. $\dfrac{50 \text{ g}}{100 \text{ mL}} = \dfrac{x \text{ g}}{450 \text{ mL}}$

b. $100x = 22{,}500$

c. $x = 225 \text{ g}$

d. $225 \text{ g} \times 3.4 \text{ kcal/g} = 765 \text{ kcal}$

Step 3: Calculate the sum of calories from the amino acids (step 1) and dextrose (step 2).
170 kcal + 765 kcal = 935 kcal

Step 4: Calculate the amount of calories from protein.
170 kcal/935 kcal × 100 = 18.2% = 18%

11. B

Step 1: Calculate the calories from the amino acids.

a. $\dfrac{8.5 \text{ g}}{100 \text{ mL}} = \dfrac{x \text{ g}}{500 \text{ mL}}$

b. $100x = 4250$

c. $x = 42.5 \text{ g}$

d. $42.5 \text{ g} \times 4 \text{ kcal/g} = 170 \text{ kcal}$

Step 2: Calculate the calories from the dextrose.

a. $\dfrac{50 \text{ g}}{100 \text{ mL}} = \dfrac{x \text{ g}}{450 \text{ mL}}$

b. $100x = 22{,}500$

c. $x = 225 \text{ g}$

d. $225 \text{ g} \times 3.4 \text{ kcal/g} = 765 \text{ kcal}$

Step 3: Calculate the sum of calories from the amino acids (step 1) and dextrose (step 2).
170 kcal + 765 kcal = 935 kcal

Step 4: Calculate the amount of calories from dextrose.
765 kcal/935 kcal × 100 = 81.8% = 82%

12. D
Step 1: Calculate how many grams of amino acids (protein) are present.

a. $\dfrac{8.5 \text{ g}}{100 \text{ mL}} = \dfrac{x \text{ g}}{500 \text{ mL}}$

b. $100x = 4250$

c. $x = 42.5 \text{ g}$

Step 2: Calculate the grams of nitrogen contained in the amino acids (protein).
42.5 g protein × 1 g nitrogen/6.25 g protein = 6.8 g nitrogen

13. B
Step 1: 190 lb × 1 kg/2.2 lb = 86.36 kg

Step 2: $76 \text{ in} \times \dfrac{2.54 \text{ cm}}{1 \text{ in}} \times \dfrac{1 \text{ m}}{100 \text{ cm}} = 1.93 \text{ m}$

Step 3: $86.36 \div 1.93^2 = 23.2$

14. C

Step 1: $\dfrac{1.1 \text{ kcal}}{1 \text{ mL}} = \dfrac{x \text{ kcal}}{320 \text{ mL}}$

Step 2: $x = 352 \text{ kcal}$

15. D
85 g × 4 kcal/g = 340 kcal

16. B
160 mL/hr × 24 hr = 3840 mL ÷ 1000 = 3.84 L

17. D
Non-protein caloric requirement = 1200 kcal × 1.4 × 1.3 = 2184 kcal

18. A
2275 kcal – 1400 kcal = 875 kcal (Note: TEE refers to the non-protein calories.)

19. C
Step 1 155 lb × 1 kg/2.2 lb = 70.45 kg
Step 2: 70.45 kg × 1.5 g/kg/day = 105.7 g/day

20. B

$$\frac{50 \text{ g}}{100 \text{ mL}} \times \frac{580 \text{ mL}}{\text{day}} \times \frac{3.4 \text{ kcal}}{1 \text{ gm}} = 986 \text{ kcal}$$

21. A

Step 1: $\dfrac{2 \text{ kcal}}{1 \text{ mL}} = \dfrac{415 \text{ kcal}}{x \text{ mL}}$

Step 2: $2x = 415$

Step 3: $x = 207.5$ mL

22. D

Step 1: $\dfrac{20 \text{ g}}{100 \text{ mL}} = \dfrac{395 \text{ g}}{x \text{ mL}}$

Step 2: $20x = 39,500$

Step 3: $x = 1975$ mL

23. A
Step 1: 210 lb × 1 kg/2.2 lb =95.45 kg
Step 2: 6'1" = 73 in × 2.54 cm/in = 185.42 cm
Step 3: BEE = 66.5 + [(13.75 × 95.45) + (5 × 185.42) - (6.76 × 71)] = 1826.08 kcal = 1826 kcal

24. B

Step 1: $\dfrac{30 \text{ g}}{100 \text{ mL}} = \dfrac{180 \text{ g}}{x \text{ mL}}$

Step 2: $30x = 18,000$

Step 3: $x = 600$ mL

25. C
Step 1: Calculate the number of milliliters of TPN the patient will receive per day.
140 mL/hr × 24 hr = 3360 mL

Step 2: Calculate how many grams of dextrose the patient will receive per day.

a. $\dfrac{25 \text{ g}}{100 \text{ mL}} = \dfrac{x \text{ g}}{3360 \text{ mL}}$

b. $100x = 84,000$

c. $x = 840$ g

SECTION 12

MISCELLANEOUS CALCULATIONS

QUESTIONS

1. Convert 43° Celsius to Fahrenheit.

    a. 27.2°F
    b. 68.1°F
    c. 87.2°F
    d. 109.4°F

2. A pharmacist measures 20.5 milliliters of alcohol instead of the desired 25 milliliters. Calculate the percent error.

    a. 9%
    b. 13%
    c. 18%
    d. 22%

3. A ferrous sulfate oral solution contains 75 mg of ferrous sulfate ($FeSO_4 \cdot 7H_2O$) per milliliter. How many milligrams of elemental iron are represented per milliliter? (Molecular weight of $FeSO_4 \cdot 7H_2O$ = 278; Atomic weight of Fe = 56)

    a. 6.7 mg
    b. 15.1 mg
    c. 22.9 mg
    d. 30.7 mg

4. The pharmacy receives an order for theophylline 500 mg IV to be dosed at 0.3 mg/kg/hr for a patient weighing 175 pounds. There is only aminophylline in stock. Calculate how many milligrams of aminophylline the patient will receive per hour.

    a. 16. 4 mg
    b. 19.1 mg
    c. 23.9 mg
    d. 29.8 mg

5. The package insert of a drug states that 5 milliliters of diluent must be added to 0.75 grams of the dry powder to make a final solution of 100 mg/mL. What is the powder volume of the vial?

    a. 2.5 mL
    b. 5.5 mL
    c. 6.5 mL
    d. 7.5 mL

6. **For a balance that has a sensitivity requirement of 8 milligrams, calculate the minimum weighable quantity that ensures a percentage of error no greater than 5%.**

   a. 63 mg
   b. 95 mg
   c. 138 mg
   d. 160 mg

7. **A patient's CBC differential reports that their white blood cell count is 9.4 × 10³ cells/mm³, segs are 52% and bands are 4%. Calculate the patient's ANC.**

   a. 5264
   b. 5830
   c. 7244
   d. 10,882

8. **Convert 67° Fahrenheit to Celsius.**

   a. 12.5°C
   b. 19.4°C
   c. 42.7°C
   d. 86.6°C

9. **A patient weighing 140 pounds requires a 5.7 mg/kg loading dose of amino-phylline. Calculate the equivalent theophylline dose in milligrams.**

   a. 290.2 mg
   b. 362.7 mg
   c. 414.9 mg
   d. 453.4 mg

10. **Calculate the percentage of sodium in sodium carbonate, Na_2CO_3. (Molecular weight of Na_2CO_3 = 106; Atomic weight of Na = 23)**

   a. 21.7%
   b. 35.1%
   c. 43.4%
   d. 46.8%

ANSWER KEY

1. D

$(43 \times 1.8) + 32 = 109.4°F$

2. C

$\dfrac{25 - 20.5}{25} \times 100 = 18\%$

3. B

Step 1: $\dfrac{278}{56} = \dfrac{75 \text{ mg}}{x \text{ mg}}$

Step 2: $278x = 4200$

Step 3: $x = 15.1$ mg

4. D

Step 1: Calculate the how many milligrams per hour the patient would receive of theophylline.

$175 \text{ lb} \times \dfrac{1 \text{ kg}}{2.2 \text{ lb}} \times \dfrac{0.3 \text{ mg}}{\text{kg/hr}} = 23.86$ mg/hr theophylline

Step 2: Calculate the equivalent aminophylline dose.
23.86 mg/hr ÷ 0.8 = 29.8 mg/hr

5. A

Step 1: $\dfrac{100 \text{ mg}}{1 \text{ mL}} = \dfrac{750 \text{ mg}}{x \text{ mL}}$

Step 2: $100x = 750$

Step 3: $x = 7.5$ mL

Step 4: 7.5 mL – 5 mL = 2.5 mL

6. D

Minimum weighable quantity $= \dfrac{8 \text{ mg} \times 100\%}{5\%} = 160$ mg

7. A

$9400 \times (0.52 + 0.04) = 5264$

8. B

$(67 - 32)/1.8 = 19.4°C$

9. A

Step 1: Calculate how many milligrams of aminophylline the patient would receive.

$140 \text{ lb} \times \dfrac{1 \text{ kg}}{2.2 \text{ lb}} \times \dfrac{5.7 \text{ mg}}{1 \text{ kg}} = 362.7$ mg aminophylline

Step 2: Calculate the equivalent theophylline dose.
362.7 mg × 0.8 = 290.2 mg

10. C

$$\frac{23 + 23}{106} \times 100 = 43.4\%$$

SECTION 13

PHARMACEUTICAL CONVERSIONS

QUESTIONS

1. 1 inch = _____ cm

    a. 1.84
    b. 2.25
    c. 2.54
    d. 3.24

2. 1 pint = _____ mL

    a. 180
    b. 473
    c. 946
    d. 1982

3. 1 gram protein = _____ kcal

    a. 4
    b. 6
    c. 8
    d. 9

4. 1 quart = _____ mL

    a. 160
    b. 245
    c. 473
    d. 946

5. 1 kilogram = _____ g

    a. 10
    b. 100
    c. 1000
    d. 10,000

6. 1 ounce (Avoirdupois) = _____ g

    a. 26.5
    b. 28.4
    c. 31.1
    d. 33.2

7. 1 tbsp = ____ mL

    a. 10
    b. 15
    c. 20
    d. 30

8. 1 fluidram = ____ mL

    a. 5
    b. 7.5
    c. 10
    d. 15

9. 1 gram fat = ____ kcal

    a. 4
    b. 6
    c. 9
    d. 10

10. 1 milliliter = ____ liter

    a. 0.0001
    b. 0.001
    c. 0.01
    d. 0.1

11. 1 grain = ____ mg

    a. 50
    b. 54
    c. 62
    d. 65

12. 1 pint = ____ cup(s)

    a. 1
    b. 2
    c. 4
    d. 8

13. 1 microgram = ____ g

   a. 0.000,001
   b. 0.001
   c. 0.01
   d. 0.1

14. 1 milliliter 20% lipid emulsion = ____ kcal

   a. 2
   b. 2.2
   c. 3
   d. 3.4

15. 1 minim = ____ mL

   a. 0.06
   b. 0.08
   c. 1.2
   d. 1.75

16. 1 tsp = ____ mL

   a. 2.5
   b. 4
   c. 5
   d. 7.5

17. 1 ounce (Apothecary) = ____ g

   a. 28.4
   b. 31.1
   c. 34.5
   d. 35.8

18. 1 gallon = ____ quarts

   a. 4
   b. 5
   c. 6
   d. 8

19. 16 fluid ounces = ____ pint(s)

    a. 0.5
    b. 1
    c. 2
    d. 4

20. 1 gram = ____ gr

    a. 12.754
    b. 13.519
    c. 14.187
    d. 15.432

21. 1 fluid ounce = ____ mL

    a. 26.7
    b. 28.5
    c. 29.6
    d. 31.1

22. 1 milliliter 10% lipid emulsion = ____ kcal

    a. 1.1
    b. 2.1
    c. 3.5
    d. 10

23. 1 kiloliter = ____ liter(s)

    a. 0.1
    b. 10
    c. 100
    d. 1000

24. 1 kg = ____ lb

    a. 2.2
    b. 2.5
    c. 2.8
    d. 3.2

25. 1 gallon = ____ mL

    a. 3025
    b. 3235
    c. 3785
    d. 3895

26. 1 deciliter = ____ liter(s)

    a. 0.1
    b. 10
    c. 100
    d. 1000

27. 1 milligram = ____ g

    a. 0.0001
    b. 0.001
    c. 0.01
    d. 0.1

28. 1 quart = ____ pints

    a. 2
    b. 4
    c. 8
    d. 10

29. 1 gram dextrose = ____ kcal

    a. 2
    b. 3.4
    c. 4
    d. 4.2

30. 1 cup = ____ oz

    a. 4
    b. 8
    c. 16
    d. 24

ANSWER KEY

1. C
1 inch = 2.54 cm

2. B
1 pint = 473 mL

3. A
1 gram protein = 4 kcal

4. D
1 quart = 946 mL

5. C
1 kilogram = 1000 g

6. B
1 ounce (Avoirdupois) = 28.4 g

7. B
1 tbsp = 15 mL

8. A
1 fluidram = 5 mL

9. C
1 gram fat = 9 kcal

10. B
1 milliliter = 0.001 liter

11. D
1 grain = 65 mg

12. B
1 pint = 2 cups

13. A
1 microgram = 0.000,001 g

14. A
1 milliliter 20% lipid emulsion = 2 kcal

15. A
1 minim = 0.06 mL

16. C
1 tsp = 5 mL

17. B
1 ounce (Apothecary) = 31.1 g

18. A
1 gallon = 4 quarts

19. B
16 fluid ounces = 1 pint

20. D
1 gram = 15.432 gr

21. C
1 fluid ounce = 29.6 mL

22. A
1 milliliter 10% lipid emulsion = 1.1 kcal

23. D
1 kiloliter = 1000 liters

24. A
1 kg = 2.2 lb

25. C
1 gallon = 3785 mL

26. A
1 deciliter = 0.1 liter

27. B
1 milligram = 0.001 g

28. A
1 quart = 2 pints

29. B
1 gram dextrose = 3.4 kcal

30. B
1 cup = 8 oz

Made in the USA
Middletown, DE
01 July 2023

34305868R00077